Practical Home
Care Medicine

D1236025

Practical Home Care Medicine

A Natural Approach

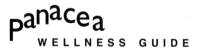

Lantern Books
A Division of Booklight Inc.

2001
Lantern Books
One Union Square West, Suite 201
New York, NY 10003

Printed in the United States of America

Library of Congress Cataloging-in-Publication Data

Murphy, Christine
Practical Home Care Medicine / Christine Murphy.
    p. cm.
ISBN 1-930051-09-3 (alk. paper)
1. Naturopathy. 2. Self-care, Health. 3. Medicine, Popular. 1. Title.

RZ440 .M86 2000
615.5'35—dc21   00-048798

"True Knowledge

works more powerfully than an inoculation.

If your knowledge of therapy and remedies is truly

imaginative or inspired—that contains a healing force. It

does not even have to be your own imagination; it can be

one you gained from another person—everyone can do this.

Fear is the opposite pole to love. If you go into a sickroom

with fear, your whole therapy has no effect. If you go in

with love, you can forget yourself and direct your whole

soul to the one to be healed. Thus, medicines and

remedies are carried by a moral element, an inner attribute

of soul and not just by virtue of their external attributes.

We are surrounded by courage on all sides, wherever we go.

If we want to live and breathe in the world, we need

courage."

Rudolf Steiner

CREDITS

"Thank you" to the many physicians, nurses and parents who shared their expertise for this book: Sandy Booth, Eileen Bristol, MT, Mary Carmichael, Wiep de Vries RN, Mark Eisen MD, Louise Frazier, Richard Fried MD, Peter Hinderberger MD, Philip Incao MD, Steven Johnson DO (tea list), Anne Creadick Kennedy RN, Alicia Landman-Reiner MD, Lioba Logan, Anna Lups MD, Nina Mihaychuk DMD, Marina Poliakoff, Elizabeth Renkert MD, Andrea Rentea MD, Charles Ridley DC ("Liver Support"), Margaret Rosenthaler RN, Cathe Sims PA, Rise Smythe-Freed RN, Jesse Stoff MD, Mary Kelly Sutton MD ("Illness" and "Herbal Teas"), and Basil Williams DO. They are commended for their continuing dedication.

Especial thanks to our dear friend Margaret Rosenthaler, RN, whose hours of careful work reviewing and adding to the present book gives it its warmth and clarity—Margaret's central theme is healing through warmth (see her article on p. 82; and the section on compresses). We are happy that her ongoing experience as a practicing nurse can be shared with all of you.

Appreciation to photographer Bonnie Nordoff and her models; the late Walther Roggenkamp, artist; editors Grace Ann Starkey, Rachel Bishop, and James Pazhavila; and artistic director James Ferguson.

Finally thanks to Mother Nature and the Weleda Company, for the incredible products listed in these pages (see Remedies, pp. 64–66, and Resources, pp. 90–91).

CONTENTS

Part One

Part Two

Part Three: Special Therapies

Notes on Part Two:
Warnings are listed in the left column, treatments in the right. Whenever a procedure recommendation is in capital letters, such as Chamomile Compress or Eucalyptus Sitz Bath, you can look it up in Part Three.

Part One

INTRODUCTION

DEAR FRIENDS,

This book is an expanded and revised edition of the magazine LILIPOH #14, "Guide to Self Care," which appeared in autumn 1998 as a special home care resource guide. The contents are compiled from the notes and experiences of anthroposophical physicians, nurses, and patients. Listed are some of their most frequently used non-prescription medicines, herb teas and kitchen remedies, and procedures. Please note that this material is not meant to replace medical advice, but rather to enhance the partnership and collaboration with your physician. It is also a work in progress, with new insights and methods constantly arising. For this reason we are leaving you a few blank pages at the end for your favorite tips, and ask that you share them with us.

May this special guide be a support to your ingenuity and courage as a healer in your own home.

And now, enjoy the knowledge that you can make a difference in the wholistic health of your family, and enjoy using this book!

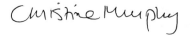

HEALING MEDICINE

The suggestions in this book are based on the following healing modalities:

Anthroposophical Medicine

A modern holistic paradigm combining homeopathy, naturopathic medicine and elements of allopathic principles. This approach, inspired by Rudolf Steiner (1864–1925) views nature, the human being, and the cosmos as related to each other, and supplements the ideas of natural (physical) science with a description of higher, non-physical, principles. The anthroposophical approach adds insight to diagnosis and healing. Many therapeutic disciplines which have been developed within this approach include: medicine, nursing, art therapy, music therapy, hydrotherapy, curative eurythmy, and massage and remedial substances.

Homeopathy

A therapeutic method inspired by Samuel Hahnemann (1755–1843) and based on the rule *similia similibus curentur* ("let likes be treated by likes"). The two elements of this tenet are the effects of drugs on the healthy body and the clinical features of disease. These two should match in symptoms, the first having been proven on healthy subjects, the second gathered from the patient's history. Homeopathy also assumes the existence of a vital (or life) force which, when stimulated by the proper substance, gives the body the possibility of healing itself.

Naturopathic Medicine

The term "naturopathy" was coined in the U.S. at the turn of the century as a combination of the terms "nature cure" and "homeopathy." The founder of naturopathy, Benedict Lust, was trained in the methods of the European nature cure movement. He added homeopathy, herbalism, and manipulation to the repertoire and instituted rigorous training standards for his method.

WHY DO WE GET SICK WHEN WE DO?

In order to be healthy we must keep an inner balance in body and soul while always moving, changing, and growing from birth to death. Although childhood is the time of most rapid growth and dramatic change, every remodeling job requires some demolition—a breaking down of part of the inherited bodily structure in order to rebuild it better. Every cold, sore throat, earache, fever and rash are indicators of the spirit's strong effort to recreate the body into a more suitable dwelling for itself. But before it can rebuild, the body must first clean up the debris, by producing mucus, pus, or a rash that work their way out or else poison the body. And just as garbage attracts vermin, so does our bodily debris attract germs. The germs don't cause the illness; they feed on it. Many remedies listed in this issue help and promote this cleansing process. Antibiotics, aspirin, and other anti-inflammatory drugs obstruct and suppress it.

Sometimes the immune system does not succeed in eliminating the body's wastes. Then the patient's inflammation may get out of control. In such cases an antibiotic is indicated. Although an antibiotic may be lifesaving, it never heals; it only suppresses the symptoms. The cause must still be healed after the antibiotic treatment, otherwise the inflammation will return, or worse, may lead to a degenerative disease.

BEFORE YOU BEGIN

1. Find a physician willing to spend a reasonable time helping you learn how to care for yourself and your family (and later be on call).
2. Begin with prevention. Create a wholesome environment in your home.
3. Have a first aid book on hand and read it through periodically *before* something happens, so that you are ready when the time comes.
4. Practice procedures such as making compresses and poultices. If possible, find an anthroposophical nurse to teach you. Practice on a family member.
5. Assemble a home remedy kit.

1 FINDING A PHYSICIAN

Although doctors these days are often looked upon with cynicism or suspicion, no task is more sacred than that of the healer. Entrusting your well-being to someone else, someone you will share your innermost hopes and fears with, is a deeply karmic matter.

Who is this person? It might be a homeopath or an anthroposophical physician, or it might simply be your neighborhood doctor who will have an ongoing relationship with you and your family, on many levels.

Finding *your* physician is definitely worth the search. Luckily you will often know it when you find the right one. Qualities that might meet you are warmth, interest, integrity, and insight, keeping in mind that no doctor knows everything and is as human as the next person.

There is nothing like collaboration for building trust, and with trust the necessity for a second or third opinion. "Shopping around," which is so devastating to a true healing relationship, can largely be avoided. You should be confident that you will have all the help and support you need to understand and learn how to take care of minor aches and pains at home.

In the end we are all in it together for the duration, learning from one another, helping one another, forgiving one another.

RESOURCES

Physicians Association of Anthroposophic Medicine (PAAM), 1923 Geddes Avenue, Ann Arbor, MI 48104. Tel: (734) 930-9462, Fax: (734) 662-1727. www.paam.net, or email paam@anthroposophy.org

American Institute of Homeopathy (AIH), 801 N. Fairfax Street, Suite 306, Alexandria, VA 22314. Tel: (703) 246-9501. www.homeopathyusa.org

2 THE HEALING ENVIRONMENT

1. Keep the bedroom clean and free of dust.
2. Arrange the bed so that light enters from the side.
3. Keep fresh, fragrant flowers visible. Remove wilted blooms daily.
4. Keep room temperature or warm fresh fluids within reach. Sipping cups are handy even for older children.
5. Put a table in reach, by the bed.
6. A communication device, like a bell or tapping stick, should be within easy reach.
7. The need for soothing images precludes the use of television, headphones, and electronically reproduced sound and visual images. The patient needs to be inwardly active, not drawn outward by external stimulation.
8. Maintain room temperature at 68–72 degrees Fahrenheit. A higher temperature may be necessary for some illnesses and for the elderly.
9. Fresh air is essential. Air the room while the patient is out (no drafts directed at the patient, please).
10. Supply a trash receptacle and empty it frequently.
11. Your good sense is the most accurate indicator of the situation.
12. The purpose is to give care. Many of your friends are caregivers also. Do not hesitate to ask for help.

FIRST AID HINTS

Keep calm. Breathe. Observe carefully. If remedies won't go down, mix them with some food or water. Always dilute alcoholic medicine in water or cool tea. In acute illnesses frequent doses of most anthroposophic remedies (every 1–2 hours) may be needed. Taking medicines in a regular rhythm is most important, but don't wake a patient to administer medicines. Keep patient reassured, warm, and as quiet as possible. Observe for changes in color, temperature, alertness, mood, and dryness (dehydration can be dangerous). Always allow him or her to rest after a compress or poultice. Serve tray meals with a damp face cloth under the plate to prevent slipping. Cover the blanket with a sheet that can be changed if it is soiled.

3 BOOKS

Healing at Home Sandra Greenstone with Clinton L. Greenstone, MD, Healing at Home Resources, PO Box 2622, Ann Arbor, MI, 48106. This book gives a broad perspective on healing at all levels and provides specific remedies and tools for promoting health. It lists a companion first aid kit, purchased separately (see page 64). 150 pp., $14.95

Caring for the Sick at Home T. van Bentheim, S. Bos, W. Visser, E. de la Houssaye, Anthroposophic Press. Basic nursing care described in detail. This book helps find meaning in illness. The first part describes the human being from the point of view of anthroposophy, and the correspondence of the plant to the body. Included are sections on pregnancy and birth, and care of the dying. 160 pp., $12.95

Home Remedies Otto Wolff, MD, Anthroposophic Press. Dr. Wolff is a family physician with many years experience. He gives practical advice on how to deal with health problems using herbal and homeopathic treatments for use at home. Natural methods resolve rather than suppress symptoms, activating the whole body and its inherent powers of healing. 96 pp., $12.95

"Overcoming Nervousness," in *Anthroposophy in Everyday Life* Rudolf Steiner, Anthroposophic Press, 1995. $12.95

First Aid Handbook Get an illustrated guide to emergency medical procedures. Join an emergency medical service or attend a course on first aid. Practice bandaging, splinting, and resuscitation with your family. Do this once a year, just as you would a fire drill. It is a wonderful feeling, knowing you are prepared and can help when needed.

RESOURCES

Anthroposophic Press, 3390 Rte 9, Hudson, NY 12534. Tel: (518) 851-2054, Fax: (800) 925-1795. service@anthropress.org / www.anthropress.org

Mercury Press, 241 Hungry Hollow Road, Chestnut Ridge, NY 10977. Tel: (845) 425-9357. fellowship@attglobal.net

4 FIRST AID SUPPLIES AND PROCEDURE

- Scissors
- Safety pins
- Band Aids, gauze, surgical tape
- Hot water bottle
- Tongue depressors
- Needle and tweezers
- Thermometer
- Bath thermometer
- Medicine dropper
- Sterile cotton balls
- Matches for sterilizing needles and tweezers
- Sterile eye wash
- Cotton swabs
- Closable (plastic) bag for ice packs
- Wool socks, knee warmers for calf or wrist wraps
- Silk scarf for sore throat
- Cotton cloth (old cotton sheets are best; rag bags are useful)
- 100% wool cloth (pieces of old blankets are a great source)
- Linen (old napkins are a good, inexpensive source)
- Two thin wool blankets
- One terry towel for compress cover
- One large towel for a body wrap

Kitchen Remedies to Keep Handy:
Sage, chamomile, ginger, horseradish, lemon, onion, honey, sea salt, frozen peas, dry mustard.

RESOURCES

Anthroposophical nurses are very familiar with compress and poultice procedures (pp. 66-78). Call the Anthroposophical Nurses Association of America (ANAA) for advice or for a nurse near you. Tel: (734) 994-8303, Fax: (734) 761-6617, or email: ANAANurses@aol.com
http://members.xoom.com/anaanurses

5 SOME COMMON FIRST AID REMEDIES

Many of these remedies are available in your local health food store. Some are available directly from the Weleda Company. Also see suggested Home Remedy Kits, pp. 64–66.

Arnica 6X (internal)	Bruises and Sprains; Muscle Pain
Arnica Essence	Bruises and Sprains
Arnica Ointment	Bruises and Sprains; Contusions; Soreness of Back; Muscle Pain
Burn Care Gel Burns;	Sunburns; Insect Bites
Calendula Essence	Skin Irritations; Mouth Sores
Calendula Ointment	Skin Irritations; Inflammations; Redness; Itching; Poorly Healing Wounds & Rashes
Carbo Betulae 3X	Stomach Cramps and Flatulence
Echinacea Comp	Severe Cold and Flu Symptom Relief
Echinadoron	Cold and Flu Symptoms; Congestion of Nose and Chest; Headache; Sore Throat
Eucalyptus Oil	For Steam Humidifier
Ferrum Phos 6X	Cold and Flu Symptoms: First Stage Relief
Infludoron	Cold and Flu: Multi-Symptom Relief
Prunus Spinosa	Fatigue; Exhaustion
Sambucus Comp	Sinusitis and Allergy Symptoms, such as Frontal Headache, Congested Head & Nose
Sedative Pilules	Sleeplessness; Nervousness and Agitation
Sinus/Allergy Pilules	Sinusitis/Allergy symptoms such as Frontal Headaches, Congested Head & Nose
Wound Care Ointment	Wounds, Cuts and Skin Abrasions.

RESOURCES

Weleda Pharmacy, Inc., 175 North Route 9W, Congers, NY 10920. Tel: (800) 241-1030, Fax: (914) 268-8574. www.weleda.com

Raphael Pharmacy, 4003 Bridge Street, Fair Oaks, CA 95628. Tel: (800) 677-0015, Fax: (916) 967-0510

American Association of Homeopathic Pharmacists, 3741 Mitford Lane, Clinton, WA 98236. Tel/Fax: (800) 478-0421

A WORD ABOUT WARMTH

The quality of warmth is little appreciated and often misunderstood. But we can't discuss health without including it. Warmth supports all healing; lack of warmth often leads to illness. Loss of warmth underlies chronic illness more often than we realize, whereas nursing the warmth maintains health in a well person and supports healing in a sick one.

As you may know, children only gradually grow into the ability to sense temperature. By age nine children usually know if they are hot or cold, but not before. As infants they are very open and vulnerable to their surrounding, losing or absorbing heat rapidly (that's why hats are recommended for use both indoors and out). The body creates physical warmth in the form of fever in an effort to rouse the immune system to action and bring the illness process to completion. The presence of fever is usually the signal of a competent immune system, as well as the activity of the organizing forces of the sick person trying to take charge in the illness situation.

We caregivers can judge an abnormality of warmth distribution simply by laying a hand—preferably warm—on hands, feet, limbs, or flanks, and comparing it with a protected area such as the tummy.

Dressing for Warmth

To dress a person well—that is for optimum health, or if there is an illness: two layers on the bottom half of the body, and three on the top are required in the cooler months of the year. There should be no gaps, the waistline tucked in so liver heat is not lost. Caps are a requirement when out of doors in cool to freezing weather. Caps or bonnets are especially important for babies and younger children, summer and winter; they protect the delicate brain enclosure from air conditioning, sun, cold, and heat, and will help prevent headaches later. The use of wool underwear in spring, winter, and fall is particularly important in strengthening the warmth organism and in giving a sense of one's own boundaries, which promotes good immune function. Children of all ages and adults should cover their feet. Wool/fleece "house shoes" are an excellent method of supporting health and should be worn in all but the hottest weather. We Americans are notoriously casual about dressing warmly, to our disadvantage in the long-term. Natural fabrics breathe best. Layer your clothing; if you sweat, one layer can be removed. The skin loses its heat to the surrounding air unless we protect it.

ARNICA Arnica montana

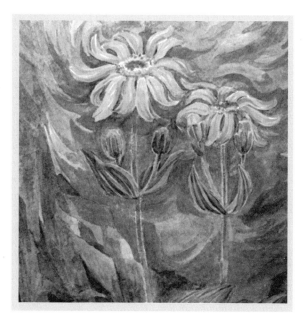

At home in crystalline heights, rooted in the moist freshness of alpine meadows, Arnica belongs to spring and early summer, to pure atmosphere and the forces of morning. The higher it grows, the more aromatic it becomes. Its vital energy derives from the massive flow of incoming sunlight at high altitudes and translates into healing forces. The body, having suffered injury, is restored, and so is the nervous system, where it is so difficult to achieve healing.

Part Two

HOME CARE GUIDE FROM A TO Z

Abscesses See boils

Abrasions_____
Scraping, injury to the skin, oozing.

Remember: deep bleeding cuts or dirty wounds need a doctor and tetanus protection.

Wash your hands! Clean abrasion well with soap and water (or just water if that is all you have). Then rinse or soak with sterile gauzes saturated with Calendula Essence diluted 1 part to 9 parts water. For a dirty abrasion it is good to soak several layers of gauze in Calendula Essence 1:10 and hold them in place with roll gauze. Leave on for several hours, remoistening with more of the Calendula/water mixture. Following these procedures apply Calendula Ointment, once or twice daily. Bandage with a sterile dressing if protection is needed.

Accident, Injury, Trauma___

Remember: Always have your first aid book in your house or car. Follow standard first aid procedures and call a physician. *Some people (1–2%) are sensitive to Arnica Essence. If you experience skin reddening or itching, stop using it.

The extent of the injury dictates the appropriateness of the remedy. Keep patient warm, quiet, and comforted. Arnica Essence is a support for any injury.* Dilute it, 1 part to 9 parts water, as a compress for bruising or as a cool compress to the forehead. Also offer Arnica 6X internal, 7 drops in water by mouth, initially every 15 minutes for shock. Follow standard first aid procedures.

Aches and Pains
See muscle stiffness, rheumatic pains

Allergies See Hay Fever

Appetite _____   Find a good recipe book. We recommend *Louise's Leaves* (see p. 85). Sometimes, if there is no active inflammatory illness and the patient is strong enough for the tub, a Nutritional Bath may be tried. (See page 69.) A walk in fresh air will also work wonders. Certain herbs, e.g., marjoram, stimulate appetite.

Athlete's Foot_____
See also Feet

Symptoms: itching, discomfort, whitish nails, scales, cracks between the toes.

Wash with Calendula Baby Soap. Put feet in a Vinegar Foot Bath. Rinse and dry well. Apply Weleda Foot Cream to dry and heal. Always treat after swimming or gym. Use Hauschka Silk Powder for cracked areas. Wear cotton, wool or silk socks and leather sandals or shoes. (see Flexible Footwear in Resources) Some Spartans say to use Weleda Mouthwash between the toes, or Thuja herb (available at health food stores) mixed with Olive Oil.

BIRCH Betula pendula

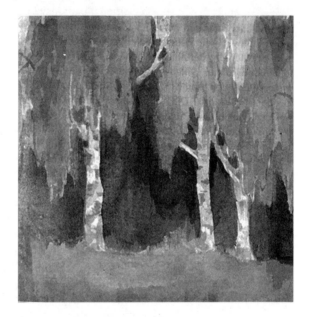

The white birch grows in northern climates in airy, light-filled groves. Birch pushes out the minerals taken up from the soil. They appear as "ash" in the characteristic white bark. The demineralized circulating liquid then rises to the leaves, giving them their youthful, light green appearance. Birch makes a wonderful spring tonic—it tends to dissolve and flush out residues.

Back Pain, Minor Strain___

Symptoms: dull muscular pain; can be caused by one-sided or excessive strain, fatigue, poor posture or faulty shoes (see Flexible Footwear in Resources).

Remember: If pain worsens or doesn't improve, see a physician.

Wear warm clothes and appropriate shoes. Use a firm mattress. Exercise (back stroke) strengthens supporting muscles. Apply a wrapped hot water bottle. Massage Arnica Massage Oil into area 2–3 times daily, or apply a Castor Oil Pack. Get Curative Eurythmy or Rhythmical Massage. The figure "B" is a good back movement. Note: Chilling a muscle may cause spasm. Apply Arnica Massage Oil or Arnica Ointment; it may stop inflammation.

Bladder Infections _____

Symptoms: burning or difficulty passing urine, bladder spasm (often in young girls), cloudy, bad-smelling urine.

Remember: Follow your doctor's instructions, especially if symptoms persist for more than a day. *****Sitz bath:** Be very cautious not to scald yourself!

Drink large amounts of fluids—at least 3 quarts a day. Uva ursi (bearberry) tea or cranberry juice are recommended, though *not together*. Avoid getting cold. This is important for prevention. People prone to urinary tract infections should not sit, unprotected, on cold surfaces. Especially, dress belly, legs, and feet warmly. Lay a wrapped hot water bottle or a Eucalyptus Oil Compress (see page 73) over the bladder. A Chamomile Steam Sitz Bath; sitting over it, not in it, may bring relief.

Boils, Abscesses _____

Symptoms: painful, tight swelling, raised red bump with pus at center.

Remember: May need lancing by a physician. Seek medical attention for abscesses that arise with fever, such that increase in size or redness, for outbreaks of multiple boils.

Apply a bulky dressing soaked in chamomile tea, as hot as can be tolerated. Or apply a dressing of raw sliced onion directly on the abcess. Reapply with fresh onion every 4–6 hours. Another very good application: is a hot soak four times daily with Calendula Essence, diluted 1:9 with water. Keep a vegetarian diet low in protein. The following can also be made into emergency compresses or plasters: mashed taro potato, onion, or whole wheat. Mouth sores: Rinse frequently with Weleda Mouthwash or Calendula Essence. A wedge of onion can also be applied here.

Bronchitis _____

Symptoms: Painful breathing, inflammation of air passages, slightly raised temperature, wheezing cough, phlegm.

Remember: Persistent cough, especially if accompanied by fever or labored breathing, may be a sign of pneumonia. Chest pains may have other causes. Observe well and report to a physician.

*Thyme can have a stimulating effect, but do not use if bronchitis is full-blown.
** Mustard, when applied properly, can often only be used *every other day.*
***Do not shower with a fever. If there is a question of pneumonia, do not put any water on the chest.

Warm feet (mustard, lemon, Sage Foot Baths). Avoid dairy and protein and increase fluids. Drink hot vegetable broth and include ginger, garlic, and onions in food. Ginger and dried thyme teas calm bronchial membranes.* Increase bowel movements. Avoid cold air. Rest. Take Anise-Pyrite 3X tablets (currently Rx only), 1 every two hours. Rub Plantago/Bronchial Balsam on upper chest and back or apply at night, as a wrap. Or make a lemon or mustard compress and apply to chest.** Put Chamomile Flowers or Eucalyptus Oil in a bowl of boiling water as a brief inhalation in a steam tent. Or simply place Eucalyptus Oil in a mixing bowl of water on the radiator or in a vaporizer. Steam from the shower can help too (don't use if the water is highly chlorinated). Turn hot water on high with the shower curtain closed. Breathe in the steam for up to 10 minutes. Then dry, wrap warmly, and go to bed.***

Bruises, Minor Bumps ____

Symptoms: subcutaneous "black and blue," swelling, soreness.

Remember: if there is intense pain or lack of movement, it could be a broken bone. Consult a physician immediately.

Start with a cool Arnica Compress (with 1 part Arnica Essence in 9 parts water) until the swelling is well controlled and begins to subside. Then proceed using Arnica Ointment, applying 2–3 times daily until blueness and soreness subside.

If there is arnica sensitivity, rub a fresh aloe leaf and spread its gel over area. Calendula is another arnica replacement. For minor head injury prepare a spray with 2 tablespoons Arnica Essence diluted with 6 oz. water. Spray scalp and hair, cover with a towel and keep covered overnight. For a bruised bone apply Arnica Essence or Comfrey compresses (comfrey is also called "knit bone"). With a fracture take Arnica 3X internally, first 10 drops hourly; then 15 drops 3 times daily for 3 days, or until the bone is healed. Keep warm!

Burn and Scalds, minor __

Symptoms: pain, redness, heat, swelling, blister formation.

Remember: For significant burns (broken skin and blistering, or loss of sensation), or if pain persists, call a physician.

Keep an Emergency handbook handy to ascertain severity of burns.

*****Note:** Extensive use of cold water can lead to cold damage. Ice cubes can lead to frostbite.

1. Immerse the burned area in cool water for 15 minutes.*
2. Keep Weleda Burn Care (Combudoron Gel) in the refrigerator for minor burns or scalds. Thickly apply over burn, and keep applying so wound doesn't stick if you bandage it. You may want to cover the gel with a cool damp compress for a while. Continue applying gel three or four times daily. Once pain and redness are gone and the skin has reformed, Calendula or Wound Care Ointment may be applied to assist complete healing. For more severe burns apply a sterilized wet wrap of boiled or purified cool water with Combudoron Liquid (1:10). It *must* remain *wet* until the pain has subsided. Then start using the Compudoron Gel as described above. Kitchen remedy: take a fresh aloe leaf, crush and apply gel to the burn. Or grate or slice a raw potato, put it on the burn and cover with gauze.

CHAMOMILE Matricaria chamomilla

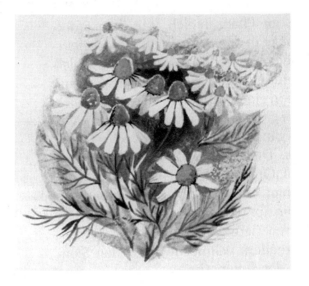

Chamomile grows from a fall rosette in light, dry places. In spring it quickly breaks into feathery yet somewhat succulent leaves. Each of the numerous long-stemmed white and golden flower heads terminate in a hollow conical receptacle holding an "air droplet." Chamomile is a salt-loving plant, which gives mastery over its otherwise sulfuric aromatic and airy nature. This allows its calming remedial qualities to unfold.

Chapped Lips, Nose _____

Chapped Lips: Weleda Calendula Baby Cream at night, Weleda Lip Balm during the day. Be sure you are drinking adequate amounts of fluid. Chapped Nose: Nasal Pommade in the nostril and Calendula Baby Cream externally.

Chest Congestion _____
See bronchitis, cough

Symptoms: tightness in breathing, hoarseness.
signs: cough, phlegm.

Remember: If there is chest pain, marked decrease in energy, loss of appetite, or trouble breathing, call your physician.

No smoking! Avoid dairy products and heavy food late at night. Go easy on protein. Eat good quality vegetable soup, radishes, cabbages, onions, spicy food such as ginger, cayenne and horseradish. Prepare a pitcher of Weleda Sytra Tea and sip frequently. Induce perspiration and reduce congestion with hot lemon tea at bedtime. Keep chest covered and warm. Don't wash in cases of acute bronchitis or pneumonia. For stubborn cases make a Mustard Plaster. Plantago Ointment on the chest is comforting (it can be covered with a 5-inch square piece of wool pinned to clothes and left on all day and all night).

Choking: Heimlich Maneuver
See First Aid Book directions

Heimlich Maneuver (learn this by heart (first aid)! People have been using the Heimlich Maneuver, named after its inventor Henry J. Heimlich, MD, to save people from choking for many decades, and now research shows its life-saving value on drowning victims as well. The Heimlich Maneuver clears the airway to the lungs, thus allowing the ventilation to be more effective. Become familiar with and practice the maneuver; it is simple to learn.

Circulation Problems _____

Remember: Coldness is often a symptom of general vulnerability. Overcoming it will increase your resistance to illness.

> "If your hands are cold, wash the dishes!"

Dress your body core warmly with wool, silk or flannel layers, warm tights or long johns, and copper insoles. Dress your children warmly, including head and neck coverings. Massage whole body with Arnica Massage Oil (Calendula Baby Oil for infants). Take a Rosemary Bath or shower. Cold hands and feet: Rosemary foot baths (1-2 capfuls in a basin of warm water) for a foot and ankle soak each morning are fantastic. Or, for cold hands try warm water and one capful of Arnica Essence for forearms, wrists, and hands. Rub Weleda Leg Toner into limbs twice daily. A Mustard Foot Bath will warm you throughout. Take brisk 10–20 minute walks 1–2 times a day. Rub children with Wala Rosemary Ointment (avoid contact with eyes). Drink nettle tea. Don't smoke.

Colds _____
Also see chest congestion, flu, sore throat

Symptoms: nasal congestion, sore throat, red or inflamed eyes.

Remember: Be sure to continue treatment for several days after symptoms disappear to prevent recurrence. Be sure you have regular bowel movements. Consult with your doctor if symptoms get "stuck" or there is excessive weakness.

A cold is an undigested external influence. If you feel one coming on, wash hands often to keep it from spreading. Dress warmly, feet too, and rest. Make a Mustard Foot Bath if you feel chilled and drink Linden Flower Tea. Take Ferrum Phos 6X. Eat nourishing food. Take Infludoron or Echinacea Compound if it feels like the flu, and drink Elderflower Tea. At night place some chamomile or eucalyptus oil in a hot steam vaporizer as an inhalation.

Cold Sores _____

Avoid fruit and regular toothpaste, chocolate, and nuts to see if causative. Excessive sweets may also be a problem.

The salt and myrrh in Weleda Salt Toothpaste or Melissa Essential Oil can be very helpful if applied topically. As a preventative: Take Mercurius Vivus 6X, 7 drops 3 times daily, when first tinglings begin (symptoms disappear). Do this for several cycles and most people will not have a recurrence. For mouth sores apply Weleda Mouthwash, undiluted, with a cotton swab.

Constipation _____

Symptoms: hard stools that are difficult to pass or inability to pass stools for three or more days.

Remember: It is vital to deal with the cause of constipation and not to rely on laxatives for any length of time. If this is habitual, a physician, evaluation may be necessary

Note: For severe or chronic cases of constipation there is nothing like a Rhythmical Massage.

Get nutritional counseling. Practice regularity. Drink a lot, but not with meals. Eat regular, small meals often, with lots of fruits and vegetables. Increase roughage. Raw carrot is excellent. Augment meals with lactic acid–fermented vegetables (sauerkraut) or fermented drinks (kvass). Avoid sugar. Have stewed prunes once daily. Epsom Salts, a teaspoon in warm lemon water in the morning, or a teaspoon of finely ground flax or psyllium seeds in yogurt are tried and proven (flaxseed must be freshly ground on the day it is used). Increase exercise. A warm Chamomile Compress will warm and relax a tight abdomen.

Convalescence _____

Remember: Use judgment before day after a fever, longer after severe illness. Realize that convalescent time is part of healing.

Blackthorn Tonic (see page 87). Drink Weleda tonics, especially blackthorn, and take Prunus or sea salt baths (1 cup to a warm tub). Eat chlorophyll-rich foods. Rest often and keep warm. Take Prunus Spinosa, 7 drops 4 times daily. Nutritional baths are helpful.

Corns _____

Soak the corn in a tea made of Chamomile. Rub gently with a pumice stone. Dry well, then apply Weleda Foot Balm.

Cough _____
Also see bronchitis, colds, flu

Symptoms: Check: Is it a "dry" cough or not? Is sputum or mucus being coughed up; what color and consistency is it? Is there pain? How frequent is the cough?

Remember: Shortness of breath, colored sputum, persistent cough with weakness, pain, fever, headache, or inability to lie flat may be pneumonia. Call the doctor.

Note: Keep feet, chest and belly warm. Don't wash the chest if pneumonia is suspected.

Increase fluids, including sips of Sytra, horsetail, chamomile, or linden teas. For children over one year and adults: Steep several large pieces of onion in one cup of honey overnight. Remove onion, add 2 tablespoons lemon juice. Sip every 3 hours. Apply Plantago Bronchial Balsam to the chest. For a dry, nonproductive cough use a chamomile tea steam inhalation (see Bronchitis), or Eucalyptus Oil in a frequently cleaned hot steam vaporizer (a cold mist or ultrasonic vaporizer could increase symptoms). Bowel cleansing and horsetail tea help prevent progression to pneumonia.

Cramps, abdominal _____
Also see menstrual cramps, premenstrual syndrome

Remember: If you don't know what the cause is, call the doctor. Physicians should approve use of heat on belly when there is pain other than menstrual cramps.

For menstrual cramps, lie down with a chamomile compress and a hot water bottle over the belly (see p. 71). For chronic menstrual cramps take Marjoram Comp (Menodoron) between periods. One dose of Melissengeist, 12 drops in a teaspoon of water, often helps.

Croup

A viral infection, which can, especially in children, lead to seal-like barking.

Remember: If breathing becomes labored or if patient becomes pale around the lips consult a physician immediately. Pneumonia and serious airway compromise are possible complications.

Bryonia 3X/Spongia 3X internally 3 times daily (see dosage, p. 63) and Plantago/Bronchial Balsam to chest. If an attack occurs at night, wrap the child in a warm comforter and take him/her out of doors. One can also turn hot water on in the shower until the bathroom is filled with warm steam. Stay there with the child until spasm loosens.

Cuts
See also wounds, dirty wounds

Remember: See doctor if the wound is too much to handle. Stitches must be done within six hours and are required if: 1. there is excessive bleeding, 2. for cosmetic reasons (face), 3. wound is gaping or located over a joint. Note that wounds are less likely to become infected if they are not stitched. Tetanus risk: Open the wound to the air while cleansing it. It may need one rinse with dilute peroxide to oxygenate it. Consult your physician regarding the need for tetanus prevention. If a wound becomes infected—increasing pain, swelling, discharge, etc.—seek medical advice.

> *"When the caregiver respects the sick person's dignity and has faith in the recovery, then the caregiver becomes like a medicine to the patient."*

Stop the bleeding. Apply pressure to cut with a clean cloth. Holding extremity higher than the heart slows bleeding. Clean well with Calendula Soap or other mild soap and water, then soak in diluted Calendula Essence. You can make a wet compress with calendula (1:10 solution in water) using sterile compresses and roll gauze to cleanse the wound and keep it moist. Leave on for several hours. Next apply Calendula Ointment as an antiseptic, and bandage. If it is a deep cut, Wound Care Ointment should be used instead of Calendula Ointment. A butterfly bandage holds a deep cut together and helps reduce scarring. Use this only if you are sure if the wound is thoroughly cleaned and rinsed one time with dilute hydrogen peroxide. Later, Wound Care Ointment will help keep scarring to a minimum.

DANDELION Taraxacum officinale

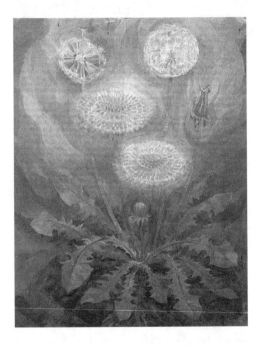

The "common" dandelion grows in all conditions with a strong tap root and leaf rosettes that vary from wide/watery to light/airy. Its bitter "milk" or latex arises in the leaves in spring, then as warmth increases, is forced back into the root. The honey-golden crown opens and closes with the sun and moves to the starry rhythms. Dandelion principally affects the fluid organization, including the stomach and the liver.

Dandruff _____

Remember: Dandruff may be a symptom of an underlying imbalance or stress-related condition. If it persists, seek advice.

* Do not use plastic with young children or infants—possibility of suffocation.

Diarrhea _____

Symptoms: frequent, watery stools, occasionally cramping after eating or drinking.

Remember: Always call the doctor for severe diarrhea, especially in infants, where there is greater danger of dehydration. Also call doctor if abdominal pain, stiffness or tenderness to touch are the main symptoms, or if you do not feel comfortable dealing with any of the procedures. Diarrhea suppressants may cause serious complications of salmonella or E-coli strains if the body can't quickly flush out toxins. Avoid them if you can.

Dry Skin _____

Remember: Physician needs to assess liver function and thyroid function.

Drink plenty of fluids and include oil in your diet. Rinse scalp with chrysanthemum tea and massage it daily. Weekly, make a warm Rosemary Hair Oil pack. Apply liberally, cover with a warm moist towel under plastic.* Keep on for 20 minutes. Then shampoo.

Sometimes a viral illness produces vomiting then diarrhea, as the body cleanses itself. Important: If there is no vomiting drink plenty of clear fluids; blueberry juice, very mild peppermint or chamomile tea, and Pedialite (1/4 tsp salt and 1 tsp sugar per 8 ounces of water). If there is vomiting, sip fennel tea. Fast: inflamed bowels heal if they have a rest from food. Then begin with clear vegetable broth or oat broth and, next day, peeled and grated apples, banana, cream of rice. Next try crackers and toast. No dairy, nuts, beans, eggs or meat until the fifth day. Take Carbo Betula 3X Powder every two hours. To minimize soreness if diarrhea is severe, wash bottom with plain water after bowel movement. If there is burning, use Calendula Baby Cream.

In spite of "fat" scares, it is vital to use plant oils such as olive or flaxseed oil in your diet. Drink lots of water. Don't bathe too often. After bathing, massage body with Arnica Massage Oil or Wild Rose Body Oil. Or apply a body oil before a warm bath or shower. Then dry briefly and immediately cover skin with an emollient to hold moisture in. Older, papery skin does well with a diluted Iris Cleansing Lotion soak.

E C H I N A C E A Augustifolia

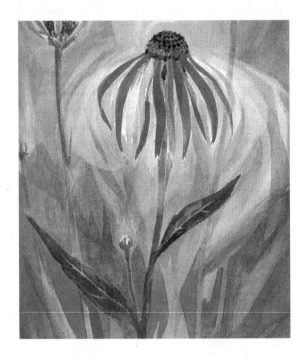

This plant is a healing gift, native to North America. Its use is for feverish and inflammatory conditions, clearly indicated by the "inflamed" flower petals. Echinacea, the purple cone flower, is a stately plant preferring dry warm places but is at home in any garden. It grows over two years, first with a leaf rosette, then rising on a long stem to its blossom.

Earache, Ear Infection____

Remember: A doctor's visit is usually required for earaches since they require a professional diagnosis. We especially recommend you contact an anthroposophical physician for the specific remedy, since ear infections can become chronic. Whatever measures you take should be in the nature of stopgap until the doctor's visit. If there is discharge or if symptoms persist for more than 36 hours, do not put anything into the ear. Call the doctor's office immediately.

Note: Not all middle ear infections require antibiotics.

If wiggling the outer ear causes pain, it is probably swimmer's ear. A dropper of vinegar in 3 tsps water 3–4 times daily, or a few drops of rubbing alcohol in the ear after swimming are first aid measures. If the pain is deep inside and not affected by wiggling the outer ear, it could be a middle ear infection, which occurs behind the eardrum and is common after colds in young children. Chamomile inhalations open the eustachian tubes and a chamomile compress soothes pain. Limit milk products. An onion poultice (p. 78) helps alleviate pain too. It also strongly stimulates the immune function to help organize the inflammation. Keep ear and head warm with a woolen cap, either alone or over the poultice. Note that complete healing takes at least 7–10 days when treating otitis media naturally. The cessation of pain is not an adequate sign. Continue with a warmed onion juice compress and a chamomile inhalation twice daily for that period.

Eyes, inflamed
See pink eye

FENNEL Foeniculum vulgare

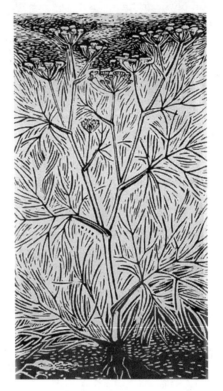

Fennel is an airy plant, with feathery leaves and a light-filled yellow umbel. Its scent and taste are mild, volatile, and sweetly fragrant. Fennel matures over two years, holding down and concentrating its growth in the first. Then, in the second year, it shoots up to fulfill its potential in the interplay of light and warmth. Fennel warms the digestive tract and acts beneficially on the air organization.

Faintness
See nausea, travel sickness

Remember: Any faintness should be noted, including its probable reason. If the condition persists, seek medical advice. If the person is warm to the touch or if there is a fever, call the physician immediatley.

Feet, Aching; Foot Blisters

Lemon or Epsom Salt foot baths soothe aching feet. For moist conditions, or tendency to blister, use Weleda Foot Cream or Tea Tree essential oil. Massage very dry feet with Weleda Skin Food. Use Arnica Massage Oil or a rosemary foot bath for warming, and diluted Calendula Essence Soak for healing blisters. Obtain properly fitting shoes (see p. 91) and wear natural fiber socks!

Fever
Also see colds and flu

Remember: Avoid giving aspirin for fever to children under 18 years. They might be susceptible to Reye's Syndrome, which can cause brain damage. Check with your physician first. Seek medical attention if the cause of the fever is unknown or if child is less than 12 months old.

Bed rest, quiet, and plenty of fluids including hot tea. Avoid protein. Horsetail tea helps the cleaning process. Induce sweating if fever is "stuck" by giving hot tea (lindenflower tea) and covering well, in addition to other measures ordered by the physician. No sponge baths if fever is high. Give lemon calf and foot wraps. If there are no abdominal symptoms, use natural measures to do bowel cleansing—three loose stools a day are ideal, even when fasting.

Flatulence, Gas

Consult a physician if this is a persistant problem and does not respond to dietary changes.

Chew food well. Review diet. Fresh dairy—milk, cottage cheese, and ice cream—are the most common causes of gas. Other foods include carbonated beverages, legumes, cabbage, brussels sprouts. In India, fennel seeds are roasted and eaten as an after-dinner digestive aid. Make a hot tea with ground ginger and honey in hot water or drink weak Triplex or fennel tea. If there is discomfort put a castor oil or chamomile compress on the tummy. Take Carbo Betula 3X, one pea-size portion at onset.

Flu _____

Symptoms: Viral flu hallmarks include fever, general muscle aches, fatigue.

Remember: Call your physician if there are other ongoing serious conditions, such as heart illness, if the immune system is weakened, if symptoms persist for more than three or four days, or if there is pain or shortness of breath. Check if there is a recent history of a deer tick bite.

Early prevention: When cold season starts, know what's "going around." Keep warm, especially the feet. Avoid "gaps" in your clothing. Massage your whole body with Arnica Massage Oil often. Eat some beets and include parsley and ginger in your diet. Drink elderberry juice or diluted extract. Take Ferrum Phos 6X.

Old Saying:
"Feed a Cold and
Starve a Fever."

At the first sign of flu or just exhaustion give hot elder flower tea. Rub entire back with Arnica Massage Oil. A relaxed sleep will usually ensue. To further minimize the flu stop eating altogether and start drinking hot herb teas and hot citrus drinks, as much as tolerated. Then keep low salt diet, plenty of liquids and rest. Drink hot lemon juice, one glass 3 times daily. Take Infludoron. A remedy that brings the body back into balance is a drink of lemon, canned (yes canned!) tomato juice, and freshly squeezed or grated garlic. All ingredients have to be mixed together. The juice can also contain other vegetables, like celery and carrots, but the tomato is essential. Empty your bowels, unless you already have diarrhea (a Dulcolax suppository works well). Try to maintain three loose stools per day, even if fasting.

For a headache caused by flu or mild fever, apply Melissengeist to the temples. Be sure you are drinking enough fluids and that your stools are loose and more frequent than usual.

If there is **no** fever, and you do not have a cardiac condition, take a hot bath or warm in a sauna or steam room. Then go to bed and sweat and sleep as long as possible. If you have a fever, just go to bed and wrap up warmly. Apply lemon calf and foot wraps. Take Ferrum Phos 6X and Echinacea Comp every four hours for a beginning feverish flu. Children under three years take Infludoron pilules that are dissolved in a teaspoon of warm water.

Food Poisoning _____
Also see diarrhea and nausea

Food poisoning usually means acute gastroenteritis.

Call the Emergency Room and your doctor immediately. If you can't reach the doctor right away, call 911.

Note: Our digestion should be able to encounter and withstand a certain amount of food adversity with impunity. To strengthen the digestive system seek wholesome food sources. Your first choice is biodynamically grown food. The second choice is organic food, and the third choice is fresh unprocessed food.

Gums _____
Also see teeth

Remember: all gum problems need a dentist's diagnosis.

Brush teeth with one drop of tea tree or fennel essential oils, or make a paste with myrrh powder, dogwood powder and/or goldenseal powder to help with bleeding gums and gum weakness. Brush with sea salt or Weleda Salt and Baking Soda toothpaste. Rinse your mouth with Calendula Essence 1:10, 30 drops echinacea tincture, or two drops of tea tree oil. Rinse immediately after eating sweet or sour food. Floss, brush, and have teeth cleaned as often as recommended by your dentist.

HAMAMELIS VIRGINIANA
Witch Hazel

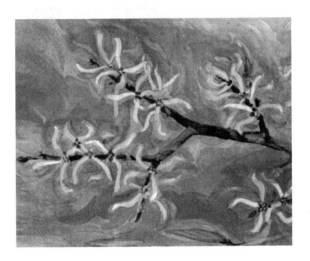

An American plant at home in light undergrowth, near stream beds. Its strong, resilient, smooth branches arch diagonally rather than rising straight towards the light. Its most unusual aspect, however, is its blossom, which occurs in early winter, when all other growth has long disappeared. This is the sign of its efficacy: bringing fluid life back to the "wintery" aspect of the skin.

Hay fever

There are anthroposophical remedies available to help with this. See your nearest anthroposophical physician.

Headache
Also see sinusitis

Symptoms: Tension headache: dull, ongoing pain that feels tight. Sinus headache: steady pain behind forehead and cheeks. Migraine headache: throbbing, nausea, visual disturbances (physician evaluation is needed for diagnosis).

Remember: Immediately contact your physician if there is vomiting, double vision, weakness, stiffness of neck, convulsions, or difficulty in swallowing

Head Cold
Also see colds, flu, sinusitis

Note: The body will always attempt to flush out what it can't digest, either through elimination or through the skin. Support this function; do not suppress it.

Sniff warm salt water or chamomile tea for temporary relief. This cleans out nasal passages and helps get rid of debris. Minimize use of foods that challenge the liver, e.g. sweets and nightshades. Go easy on protein. Don't rub the eyes! Take sinus/allergy formula.

Hot rosemary bath foot soaks often bring relief. At the first sign of migraine put feet into a mustard foot bath (p. 75), then go to bed in a dark room. Dab Melissengeist or Arnica Essence on the temples. Make an ice pack on the forehead and hot pack on the neck. Sometimes bitter teas help. Peppermint/lavender flower essence blended in the vaporizer or on the temples is very good for nervous/stress headache, as is peppermint tea, or munching a leaf of feverfew.

Eucalyptus oil in a hot steam vaporizer for room humidity at night. Chamomile tea steam inhalation 1–4 times daily. Melissengeist to the temples. Make sure bowels are moving. For swollen glands in the neck gently massage Archangelica Ointment into the area 2–3 times daily. Weleda Nasal Pommade clears nasal passages and protects the nose. Be sure lower body is very warm. Mustard foot baths may help.

Heat Rash

Also see dry skin

Dust skin with cornstarch, or Weleda Baby Powder. Take a warm Aveeno (oatmeal) bath. Apply aloe gel or Weleda Diaper Care Cream.

Hemorrhoids, Minor

Also see constipation

Remember: any home measures are stop-gap. Look to a physician for advice on long term care of hemorrhoids.

Prevention: Avoid straining at bowel movements. Drink more fluids if stools are hard. Get nutritional counseling. Keep a high-fiber diet (fruits and vegetables). Apply witch hazel salve, Wound Care Ointment, or Calendula Ointment twice daily, or St. John's Wort Oil or Aloe Vera Gel. Prepare an Oak Bark Tea Sitz Bath. (This should not be done in a pan that contains iron—use glass or enamel/porcelain.) Soak oak bark overnight (one heaping tablespoon in 3–4 cups water), then boil until extract has a dark color.

Hoarseness

Remember: Hoarseness that lasts longer than a week, or is not explainable by circumstances should be reported to your doctor.

Drink hot lemonade or ginger tea with honey. The "onion" treatment described under "Cough" is worth the effort if it's a stubborn case and you are committed to getting rid of it quickly. Gargle with warm Weleda Mouthwash or salt water. Put Calendula/Cepa/Mercurialis Ointment on throat and wear a silk scarf. Take Cinnabar 6X, 3 times daily. Give your voice a rest. Anise Pyrite 3X (available by prescription) is very helpful.

IRIS Iris Germanica

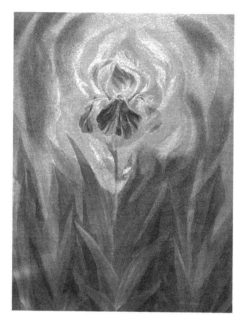

Like the rainbow, the beloved iris combines the natural forces of water and light in an unusually powerful way. It can adapt to extreme dryness or moisture because its rhizomes, stalks, and leaves have special layers that protect them. The top of each new leaf looks as though it were covered with dew, but these droplets come from inside the plant, secreted through special cracks, giving each leaf its own moist micro-climate, keeping it smooth and soft. Interestingly, the ability to retain water makes iris a homeopathic remedy for migraine, the head pain caused by pressure of excess fluid to the brain's blood vessels.

Indigestion, heartburn ___

Remember: If condition persists seek medical advice.

Parsley, parsley, parsley! Make a weak fennel tea, or drink a mix of ground ginger and honey in hot water.

Influenza See flu

Insect Bites and Stings __
Also see tick bites

Scrape stinger off the surface of the skin (don't squeeze: flick). Apply burn gel (Combudoron), Aloe gel, or a cut onion as soon as possible. Weleda Calendula Toothpaste over bite draws toxins and reduces inflammation. A baking soda paste is especially good for bee stings. If you're going outside, chew a plantain leaf soft and apply it!

Insect in Ear _____

*Remember:** Don't shake a baby —move head back and forth. Go to the physician's office to have the insect removed if it does not come out easily.

A few drops of olive oil or other cooking oil placed in the ear will kill the insect. Remove with tweezers only if you can see it, otherwise tip head and have the person shake his or her head gently.*

Insomnia _____
Also see stress

Remember: If this is more than a passing condition it may be the sign of underlying disharmony or illness and needs the attention of a physician.

Note: Prepare for going to bed as if going on a trip—it is a real process that needs care and attention.

Sonio, chamomile, or other herbal tea, toast and honey, or warm milk and honey, at bedtime, because warmth and sweets help trigger the snooze response. No TV! No caffeine and no chocolate! Review your day backwards when you come to rest. Diffuse Lavender Essential Oil in your bedroom. Take a warm lavender bath at bedtime. Take Weleda Sedative Pilules or Avena Sativa Comp, especially when on a trip with a time shift.

Itching _____
Also see dry skin, heat rash, insect bites and stings

Ascertain the cause! Could it be lice? Avoid excessive showering and bathing. Two times per week in winter is generally enough.

LAVENDER Lavandula officinalis

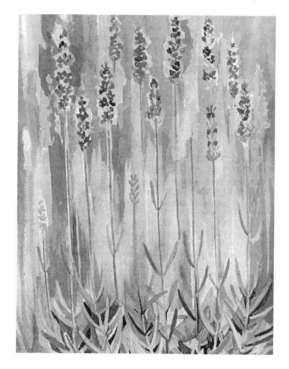

Lavender, this noble plant, basks in dry, warm Mediterranean fields. Its long, elegant stems rise from a supporting woody bush, allowing dreamlike flowers to unfold their pure aroma closer to the sun and farther from the earth. This is the image of sleep, tethered but rising out of the body into a pure distillate of light and warmth. Lavender has a calming, digestive effect; it allows the ego to uncramp.

Jet lag _____

Note: Your physician might prescribe Cardiodoron

A few days before traveling adjust your rhythms to the new time. Move meals accordingly. Drink plenty of fluids, especially water, but no alcohol. Bring your own water along. As soon as you arrive, make the most of daylight. Go out at noon and look at the sky. Try not to sleep until the bedtime hour of that place.

Kidney Pain _____

Remember: Your doctor should be consulted promptly.

Note: many people confuse lower back pain with the kidneys which are located at and below the level of the lowest ribs at the back.

Keep area warm and protected. Drink plenty of warm fluids such as horsetail tea, cranberry juice or cranberry concentrate, diluted in water. Always keep the kidneys warm. Among other reasons: The kidneys are easily damaged by cold. Avoid refrigerated drinks.

Laryngitis _____
Also see cough, hoarseness, sore throat

Apply Calendula/Cepa/Mercurialis Ointment to the neck. Make a chamomile inhalation, and sip sage tea with honey. Keep throat wrapped in a silk scarf, or one of wool in the winter.

Supporting the Liver. Cleansing drinks: dandelion leaves or parsley leaves tea or one fresh lemon in a cup of warm water. **Food that helps cleanse the liver:** endive, garlic, cucumbers, artichokes, beets with their greens, papaya. **Self-care:** Gently massage the liver area just over the lower front right rib cage with St. John's Wort Oil for one to two minutes. **Yarrow compress:** See page 74.
Exercise to help gently decongest the liver: Bend at the waist and gently rotate from the waist in a clockwise direction for twelve revolutions, twice a day. **Soul exercises, observation:** Practice observing an object for five minutes in every detail. Mentally describe the size, shape, color, texture, and so on, just as it appears to your gaze. Do this every morning.

MARIGOLD Calendula officinalis

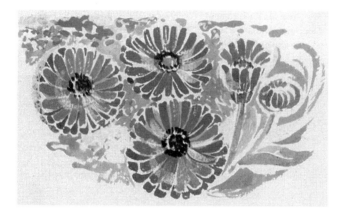

This sturdy medieval plant is as happy in country gardens as it is in refuse dumps. Its strong, ungainly, proliferating growth culminates in symmetrical golden flowers that quickly fade and are replaced by budding flowers all summer long. Calendula is a visible example of the transition from watery chaos to the sun-like qualities of form, light, and warmth—qualities that are needed to cleanse and heal a wound.

Menstrual Cramps _____
see cramps

Frequent small meals (try barrel, cured organic sauerkraut). No raw vegetables or grains during menses. Prepare a bitter tea and sip with lemon or lime throughout day. Ginger tea, chamomile tea, or raspberry leaf tea are also useful. Keep bowels moving. Stay warm, especially in the lower body. Try a Chamomile Abdominal Compress if you know your diagnosis, or apply Oxalis Ointment to lower abdomen. Use Weleda Marjoram Comp when not menstruating. Melissengeist, 12 drops in a teaspoon of water is helpful.

Morning Sickness _____

Have dried crackers at bedside to eat before rising. Eat a little food every two hours. Drink a good quality ginger ale or ginger tea.

Motion Sickness _____
Also see nausea

Acupuncture wrist bands. If you can, do the driving—drivers rarely get sick: they have their eyes fixed on the road. If you can't drive, put 7 Aurum/Valeriana Pilules under the tongue every few hours as needed.

Mouth Ulcers _____

Remember: Consult a physician if condition persists.

Rinse frequently with diluted Calendula Essence or Weleda Mouthwash. Floss. Check general state of health. Avoid acid foods and excessive sweets.

Muscle stiffness _____
Also see rheumatic pains

Remember: If pain becomes acute, consult a physician. For cramps in the calves which occur with ambulation, consult a physician.

Apply Arnica Massage Oil (birch, lavender, arnica, and rosemary) after exertion. Weleda Arnica Ointment massaged into smaller area. Take a rosemary bath. For leg cramps: leg toner (contains copper). Apply gently—don't rub calves hard. Drink birch tonic or tea. Dress warmly.

NETTLE Urtica dioica

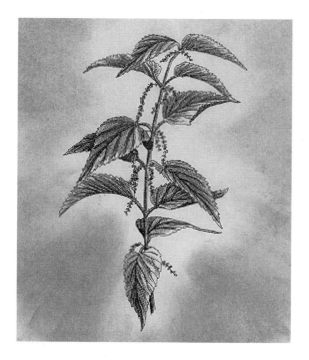

Young nettles are as good to eat as spinach. They nourish the earth as well. Their hot sting, developing as they mature, tells you: "Do not disturb" in this important work. Nettle is mostly leaf, breathing and binding water to air in its rhythmic, spiraling growth—transforming both into an abundance of chlorophyll and fiery iron. Its signature is that it cures what it causes— scalds, burns, sunburns, and insect stings (as in Weleda Burn Care).

Nasal Congestion _____
Also see head cold, flu

Remember: Small children should be monitored for ease of breathing and may need suctioning by a physician. *No spicy foods for babies! No swabs in baby's nose.

*Spicy foods (ginger, cayenne, horseradish) make nose and eyes run and help clear congestion. Cloves and hot peppers are expectorants. For blocked nasal passages apply Nasal Pommade or Plantain Ointment on the rim of the nostril, also massaged into sinus areas beside nose and eyebrows, and at base of skull. Use a hot steam vaporizer with eucalyptus essential oil, especially at night, or chamomile inhalations.

Nausea, Travel Sickness _
Also see faintness, dizziness

Leave stomach empty for 6 hours before traveling. Nux Vomica 3X, 10-12 drops before travel, or every 2 hours as needed. Melissengeist, 15 drops in water every 2 hours, increasing time between doses as condition improves. Take ground ginger tea, begin 3 hours before trip. When driving, stop every 2 hours to exercise and take a small snack. Chamomile or peppermint tea soothe stomach. Wear acupressure wrist bands.

Nervousness, Restlessness

Note: A physician may prescribe Cardiodoron or other remedies.

Come to inner rest three times a day if possible. Read *Overcoming Nervousness* (see page 11). Exercise in the fresh air. Avoid media. Take a pine bath (regularizes breathing) or a lavender bath or foot bath in the evening. Drink Sonio tea or lavender tea. Take 7–10 Sedative Pilules or Aurum/Valeriana Comp.

Nose bleeds _____

Lie back and pinch nostrils firmly together until bleeding stops. An Arnica compress over the bridge of the nose may help. Prevention: a humidifier (not ultrasonic). Calendula Ointment or Nasal Pommade on the rim of the nostrils at night.

PRUNUS SPINOSA Blackthorn

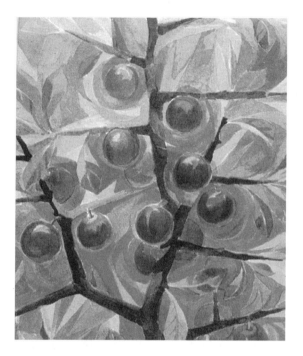

Tremendous strength resides in this thorny
wayside bush whose tough branches yield the
solid Irish shillelagh. It is one of the first to
flower in spring, with delicate blossoms covering
the bark. Then it leafs abundantly, slowly
developing a fruit which does not ripen until the
first frost. Blackthorn stores concentrated
upbuilding spring and summer forces. It is often
given as a tonic after illness.

Operations _____

Remember: This advice is in conjunction with other preparatory procedures and in collaboration with your physician only. Your anthroposophical physician can also prescribe more specific remedies.

Take Arnica 6X one week before and two weeks after surgery. Allow adequate convalescent time. Rest and keep warm. Drink Blackthorn Tonic. Apply Wala Moor Lavender Oil to chest as a protective measure. Avoid use of media for entertainment. TV especially draws on forces you need for healing. Drink adequate fluids and maintain a nutritious diet.

Pink Eye, Inflamed Eye __

Remember: This can be viral or bacterial. A sticky yellow discharge of the eyelids is usual. Always consult a physician especially if it persists more than 3 days, or immediately if there is eye pain or light sensitivity, if the eyelids get red and hot, if there is fever, or if eyesight is cloudy or impaired.

Wash hands often. Everything you touch to the eye (like a compress) should be thrown away. Keep nasal passages clear. Frequent warm compresses using diluted eyebright, chamomile, calendula, or fennel will clear most infections. Try a chamomile steam. Drink horsetail tea. Rest the eyes.

Poisons _____

Note: Keep the number of your local **Poison Control Center** prominently posted in your house and handy in your car. Call there first, then call 911.

Treat all medicines with respect. Even homeopathic medicines should be kept out of the reach of children. While most of them are non-toxic, there are exceptions. Separate external medicines from oral so that one is not inadvertently mistaken for the other. **Always read labels. Always lock your medicine cabinet.**

Premenstrual Syndrome __
Also see menstrual cramps

Drink Melissa tea 1/2 cup twice daily. For long-term treatment: Weleda Marjoram Comp (Menodoron) 15 drops 3 times daily, except during period for at least 3 months. Take vitamin E and Evening Primrose Oil. Regular exercise is very helpful.

ROSEMARY Rosmarinus officinalis

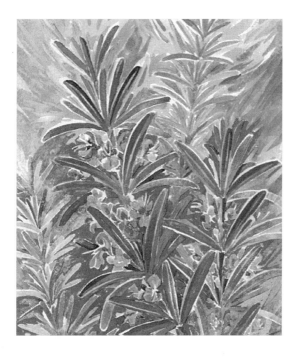

A woody bush that loves the sun, wind and sea, rosemary draws warmth and light into itself so forcefully that each leaf becomes a "flower" full of spicy fragrance, while the tiny flowers themselves remain insignificant, blossoming close to the stem. Yet the fiery, needlelike leaves are full of salt as well, so this plant is like a smelling salt—it calls forth consciousness, memory, the warmth of courage, and the will to heal.

Rheumatic Pains _____

Symptoms: pain in the joints, especially in the morning, stiffness, muscle pain, loss of function, swelling.

Remember: This can be due to many causes such as metabolic disturbances, degenerative processes, infections, or chronic inner distress. Your physician should diagnose the illness.

Keep warm—no "cold spots." Wear copper. Exercise. Rhythmical Massage and Therapeutic Eurythmy are very effective. Keep a balanced, low-meat, diet. Some people find avoiding nightshades (potatoes, tomatoes, peppers, eggplant, etc.) helpful. Apply Arnica Ointment locally 2 times daily. Cover with a wool or flannel cloth. You can also rub your whole body with Arnica Massage Oil after showering or use it to warm and loosen the afflicted area, if not inflamed. Rheumadoron Ointment, applied externally, is often helpful.

Rashes, Itches, Poison Ivy

Symptoms: redness, itching, blistering, oozing or scaling and pain.

Remember: Treat the same as burns. Get help when in doubt.

Apply burn care gel for cooling, soothing, and healing. Calendula (Rash Care) Ointment or Aloe gel help too. Internally this combination is very good: Rhus Tox 6X/Betula Cortex 10X, 10 drops 3 times daily. For poison ivy: Wash with a pine tar soap, make tepid oak bark tea compresses. Encourage bowel elimination. Drink extra water. Go easy on protein.

Poison Ivy, Poison Oak, Poison Sumac

Poison Ivy and Oak are found practically anywhere in the United States and southern Canada (Poison Ivy more on the East Coast, Poison Oak on the West). Poison Ivy (Rhus toxicodendron) has three shiny leaves with greenish flowers and whitish berries. Poison Oak (Rhus radicans) is a shrub with three-leafed clusters, resembling that of an oak leaf. Poison Sumac grows as a shrub or small tree and is found in swampy areas of the eastern half of the United States and Canada. The leaves are smooth-edged, pointed, and range in odd numbers anywhere from seven to thirteen.

SAMBUCUS NIGER Elder

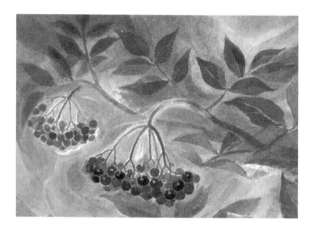

An ancient American plant, it provided a home for the good spirits of the house as legend would have it. The elder blossoms profusely with large, yellowy-white umbel clusters, each umbel composed of numerous small aromatic flowers. In autumn the clusters grow heavy with potent dark berries. Their juice has always been popular as a warming drink, good for colds, or as a cold preventative.

Scars

Wound Care Ointment or Vitamin E Capsules twice a day, until healed. Protect the wound and the healing scar from the sun to decrease the amount of melanin at the site.

Shock, Trauma
Also see Accident

Arnica 6X 1-7 drops every 2 hours for a few days for shock (accidents, falls, minor head trauma, etc.) **Keep warm!** Chamomile Abdominal Wrap appropriate in cases of emotional shock or trauma.

Sinusitis

Symptoms: cheek pain and/or pain in forehead, fullness in the sinuses, and sometimes pain in the teeth (referred pain).

Remember: Seek help if inflammation develops around eyes, if improvement does not occur in a week, or if relapse occurs within a year.

Avoid dairy! Sniff salt water or warm weak Lemon Balm tea as an antiviral. Lightly rub Calendula/Cepa/Mercurialis Ointment or Nasal Pommade on skin over sinuses, or a Horseradish/Sinus Compress for older children or adults. Take a Rosemary Foot Bath. Drink Elder Tonic. Internally: Sinus/Allergy Formula (Sambucus Comp). Be especially attentive to keeping your whole lower body and feet warm. Wool tights are a good idea.

Skin see dry skin

Sore Throat
Also see swollen glands

Remember: Sore throat accompanied by fever or swollen glands may signify a strep infection. It should be seen by the doctor, especially in children up to 15 years old.

Drink Sage Tea or Sytra Tea. Gargle with warm salt water, Calendula Essence, or Weleda Mouthwash. Suck on a clove. Try a warm potato compress on the neck or a raw onion poultice, warmed with a hot water bottle and bound to the neck. Archangelica or Mercurialis/Calendula/Cepa Ointments are effective. Take Cinnabar Comp. Mainly, keep neck well covered, preferably with a silk scarf. Drink plenty of liquids and keep bowels loose.

Splinters/ Foreign Bodies

Remember: If in doubt see a physician immediately; and always for embedded objects in the eye. For treatment of larger embedded foreign bodies see your first aid book!

Keep a good-quality splinter removal kit at home. Soak area in diluted Calendula Essence before removing splinter. Sterilize all instruments (needle/tweezers) for 10 minutes in boiling water or heat in a flame. Wipe with sterile gauze or cotton ball.

Sprains and Strains _____
Also see tendonitis

Symptoms: pain, swelling, difficulty moving joint, bruising.

Remember: Do not massage or heat an acutely injured area in the first 24 hours. See a physician if pain is severe and mobility very limited, to assess possibility of a fracture.

Use diluted Arnica Essence (1:10 solution) as a wet compress or Arnica Ointment, 3–4 times daily, or Arnica Massage Oil if that's all you have. Protect area and keep it quiet. Elevate a limb. Give Arnica 3X, 7 drops by mouth. Knee injuries: Avoid fats in diet temporarily. This is associated with the gall bladder in relation to the knee and speeds healing.

Stage Fright, Fears _____

Take 7–10 Sedative Pilules (Avena Sativa), three times daily.

Stings _____
Also see insect bites, stings, and tickbites

Remember: Don't pinch with tweezers. Can cause more venom to be released. Be aware of poisonous insects in your local area.

Scrape stinger off the surface of the skin (don't squeeze or pluck out). Apply Aloe Gel or Combudoron Gel (Burn Care). An outdoor quick-fix: sugar applied to mosquito bites. Jellyfish stings: Ammonia or alcohol will neutralize the poison. Dilute 1 to 4 with fresh water for a bath or soak.

Stomach Ache _____

Remember: Abdominal complaints should be assessed by a physician.

A chamomile compress and chamomile tea can bring relief. A chamomile compress may be used if your physician approves the use of a hot application for this condition. Take Chamomile 3X three times daily.

Stress _____
Also see tension, nervousness, restlessness

Introduce rhythm to the day, with regular meals, a set bedtime, and plenty of exercise and relaxation time. Avoid stimulating foods and drinks such as spices, coffee, tea. Drink Sonio tea at night. Avoid activities that overstimulate the nervous system. A long walk in nature each day is beneficial. Attentively observe your surroundings. A warm lavender bath at night assists sleep. Arnica Massage Oil in nape of neck moves consciousness to the sleep pole. Sedative Pilules help for nervousness. Melissengeist can be used as smelling salts, patted on forehead for headache, or internally for emotional disturbances. Be sure your feet are warm. Provide at least for short regular periods of inner quiet and reflection.

Sunburn _____

Remember: Try to avoid sunburn. Use a good sunscreen (preferably one using natural substances).

Cover burn with Burn Care Gel to cool and protect. Keep applying 3–4 times daily. Once the pain and redness have gone and the skin has reformed, Wala Wund and Brand Gel or Calendula Ointment can be applied to assist complete healing. Kitchen remedy: To alleviate pain, put a cup of vinegar into the bath and bathe in it, or mix some vinegar with water for a compress.

Swollen Glands _____

Remember: Check for cause with physician.

Archangelica Ointment, gently applied to the neck 2–3 times daily, is often used. Wrap neck with flannel if glands there are affected.

Teeth

Remember: If there's a sudden toothache, call the dentist. Massage oil of cloves into the area as a first aid measure, or apply onion as described.

Prevention of tooth decay in childhood

Tooth decay is countered by strengthening the etheric life forces. Rudolf Steiner gave medical students a formula in 1920. Take Chlorophyll Ointment 1% made from nettles high in iron and silica. Rub it into the child's lower abdomen at bedtime, from the belly button downward. Nina Mihaychuk, DMD says: "It is a very simple thing; something I would send home in every mother's baby pack." Start after one year at the latest, or when the primary teeth are out. The only drawback is that the pajamas may get stained green.

Weleda Mouthwash for gum maintenance after each brushing. Its ingredients, myrrh and ratanhia, are bitter substances that draw together the tissue of this most watery realm. Weleda Salt Toothpaste is very helpful. For gum inflammation or toothaches: Cut a piece out of a layer of a strong yellow onion, leaving the membranes intact. Slide it into the pocket between the gum and the cheek. Change every hour. Remove onion before going to sleep. An old Russian household remedy says to take pure olive oil into the mouth, holding for 20 minutes. Then spit out completely, rinse, and brush away residue. This seems to increase the health and resistance of teeth and gums. Dental abscesses: Rinse with warm diluted Calendula Essence. Before and after bone surgery (surgical endodontics) take Arnica 6X internally, 7 drops 1/2 hour before, and every hour after, for one day. To help stop gums bleeding: Use a black tea bag instead of gauze because of the beneficial qualities of the tannic acid.

Tendonitis, Tennis Elbow
Also see sprains and strains

Take 7 drops Arnica 3X orally and apply Arnica Ointment topically to area. Rest the limb.

Tickbites

Remember: Remove as soon as possible to avoid likelihood of Lyme Disease. If tick is deeply imbedded and won't come out. get help from a physician. Any rash, joint pain, or flu-like symptoms within 4 weeks of a deer tick bite should be investigated by a doctor.

Tickle the underbody of the tick. Try to grasp it with fine tweezers as close to the skin as possible without squeezing its body. Be sure to get all of it out. Wash with soap and water. Put a piece of onion over the lesion and tether with a Band Aid. It has a drawing effect and increases the immune response. You may take Echinacea Comp and Ferrum Phos 6X as a preventative.

Tiredness, Trouble Waking

A face wash with Rosemary Soap each morning, or a rosemary rath with warm water, or a rosemary bath splashed on your washcloth for the shower can bring instant awakening. A rosemary foot bath is very helpful for elderly people.

Travel Sickness
Also see faintness, nausea, jet lag

Nux Vomica 3X daily 10–12 times in water as needed.

Urinary Tract Disturbance

Remember: See a physician first.
*Do not drink cranberry at the same time as bearberry as it negates the effectiveness of the bearberry.

Drink 2–3 quarts of water or other fluids a day if tolerated. Bearberry leaf tea (Uva ursi) helps flush urinary system when infected.* Drink 2–3 times daily. Avoid caffeine. Keep warm, especially lower body from waist down, and feet. Apply a eucalyptus or St.John's Wort oil compress over the lower abdomen.

VIOLA TRICOLOR Wild Pansy

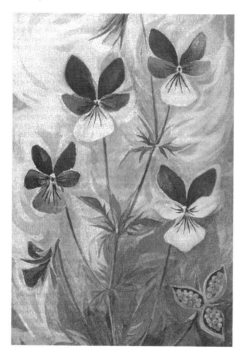

Traditionally, Wild Pansy loved growing in or near grain fields. Although modern chemical agricultural has largely displaced it there, this sympathetic plant still finds many corners in which to flourish. Its insignia is its mercurial ability for change, as seen in the individual "faces" of its blossoms. Yet it is also steadfast and uniformly tenacious in its root growth. Folk medicine has often used it as a remedy for skin conditions.

Vaginal Itching _____
Also see yeast infection

Remember: See a physician if problem persists.

Calendula Essence, 1 tsp to a cup of warm water as a cleansing douche. Use Calendula Baby Cream for dryness.

Varicose Veins _____

Apply Weleda Leg Toner to legs twice a day and elevate feet. No prolonged standing. Wear support hose. Rosemary lotion works topically as does horse chestnut herbal extract. Increase exercise. Give special care to the liver.

Vomiting _____
Also See nausea

Remember: A physician must be seen for projectile vomiting, for signs of dehydration, and for vomiting after a blow to the head, or if the condition is not promptly resolved with this treatment. For instance, under one year of age, seek physician's advice.

This is often a way for the body to eliminate indigestible or unwanted substances. It can occur easily, especially in infants. Evaluate for dehydration. Give Nux Vomica 3X, 10–12 drops every 2 hours. Initially start with a fast, giving chamomile tea, 1 tsp every 15 minutes, gradually increasing the amount. Prepare about 3 loose organic chamomile flowers to 1 cup boiling water. Cover and steep 1 minute, then strain. If vomiting has stopped, slowly start oat broth. Next day give puffed rice crackers, grated apple, cream of rice and vegetable broth. Next day you may start giving soft cooked foods. If vomiting restarts, go back to fasting and chamomile tea.

WILLOW Salix alba

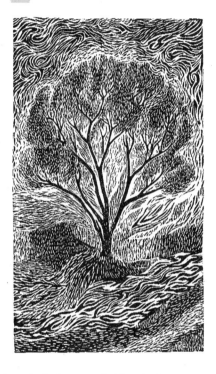

This tree truly forms a bridge between water
and air. It grows in moderate to cold zones,
following rivers and streams, drawing quantities
of water into its roots and soft, malleable
branches. Willow has always been used for
feverish colds with rheumatic pains; its salicylic
acid was used for aspirin when it was first
produced. Anthroposophical medicine uses
willow leaves to normalize intestinal function
and willow bark for chronic diarrhea.

Warts

Remember: Check, and if necessary, treat digestion.

Soak until skin is soft. Dry. Apply Thuja Ointment, cover with salt and a Band Aid overnight; six weeks if necessary. Feet must be warm and dry.

Worms

Remember: These measures are to be taken in collaboration with your doctor.

For a small child mince one clove of garlic, mix with a tsp of honey and give at bedtime. Increase dosage for older children. Treatment can be repeated in three days. For pinworms: Eat grated raw carrots; just that! A flower essence parasite cleanse (Garlic Essence) helps in certain cases.

Wounds
Also see cuts

Remember: Seek medical assistance if area becomes increasingly red, swollen, painful, etc.

Keep wound clean and rinsed with diluted (1:10) Calendula Essence. Cover with Wound Care Ointment or Calendula/Cepa/Mercurialis Ointment to lesion twice daily. All are excellent healers.

Whooping Cough (Pertussis)

Whooping Cough is extremely infectious from the start of the coughing till about four weeks later, and in rare cases, six weeks. More than half of the children who attract whooping cough are under two years old. Keeping your child isolated at home is important to prevent infection in other children. Consult with your physician throughout.

Advice for Parents

Handle the situation calmly and gently. Be patient and supportive. Gently encourage the child to breathe in and cough again during the spasm. Provide rest, comfort, and consolation. Avoid sedatives and cough-suppressants (the cough would become less frequent and strong, causing mucus to remain in the lung and possibly resulting in pneumonia or a lack of oxygen to the brain). Provide a quiet environment and avoid stimulating sense impressions as much as you can. Wrap the child up warmly in bed and give warm drinks such as hot linden tea. Anthroposophic prescription remedies can be very helpful.

YARROW *Achillea millefolium*

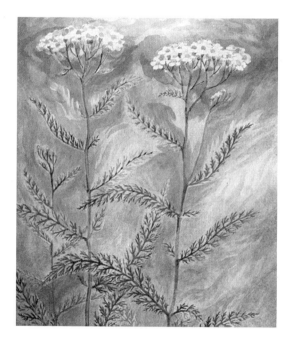

The hardy yarrow loves dry heights. From the first its leaves are so fine and aromatic that flowers are expected, but leafing continues into high summer, culminating in the spicy umbel, which blooms well into fall. This slow development allows full absorption and maturing of the seasons' elements, blending earthly salt with silica and sulfur. Yarrow is warming and healing to digestion and to the blood.

Yeast Infection, vaginal __

Remember: Ask your physician what the underlying causes may be.

Note: Wear loose-fitting clothing and pure cotton or silk panties. Boil all undergarments. There are anthroposophical remedies available on prescription which are very helpful.

Avoid sweets; there is often a carbohydrate intolerance/weak digestion. Avoid bubble baths and too much soap; they cause irritation. Use a diluted Calendula Essence douche: 1 part to 9 parts warm water, or a hot eucalyptus sitz bath. To prepare this bath, fill a small bottle or jar 1/3 with water. Put 1–2 capfuls of eucalyptus essential oil in the jar and shake vigorously to disperse it in the water. Draw the bath as warm as tolerated and as high as the navel and pour the oil mixture into the running water. After the oil and water mixture is added, enter the bath. Sit for about 15 minutes with a towel over the shoulders (you should never sit in cool water!). Don't use soap. After bath, dry off very carefully, wrap warmly and rest for 30–45 minutes (may be done at bedtime). Use Calendula Baby Cream for external irritation.

You may also try a vinegar sitz bath: Add 1 tbsp vinegar to 1/2 tub warm water. Sit in for 15–20 minutes. Dry off very carefully—you might even use a hair dryer on a low setting.

Part Three

SPECIAL
THERAPIES

INTERNAL REMEDY DOSAGES

No two individuals experience an illness in exactly the same way and, as a rule, homeopathic medicines are individually prescribed. Some medicines, however, serve a wider spectrum of common acute ailments such as the ones found in these pages. They are over-the-counter remedies and are usually given 3 times a day, 15 minutes before meals.

Remedies should be given regularly and consistently if they are to work, but don't wake an ill person to give a remedy—sleep is the best healer. As the illness improves, the frequency of the dose can be decreased from every 1 or 2 hours to 3 or 4 times daily, but do not stop the remedies until 2 or 3 days after the illness is gone, or after the other symptoms have cleared up.

The "X" or "D" after a medicine is the symbol for a homeopathic potency. 1X, or D1, for example, means that one part medication has been rhythmically combined with 9 parts carrier substance to a potency in the first degree. 2X means that one part of the 1X has been rhythmically combined with a further 9 parts carrier substance.

General Instructions for Use of the Remedies

Tablets: 1 tablet 3 times a day.

Powders: A little heap of powder the size of a green pea, on a tip of a spoon.

Pellets, or Pilules: Figure dosage by the age of the patient. For example, 3 years=3 pellets. From age 7 the adult dose of 7–10 pellets is usually given.

Liquid Remedies: Give liquid remedies in a teaspoon of water, preferably on an empty stomach, 7 drops 3 times a day, or as stated on the label. For infants under 6 months use one drop. Use 2 drops from 6 months to 2 years and after that as many drops as the child's age in years (4 years old, 4 drops, etc.). Over 12 years old and adults use 7 drops.

SUGGESTIONS FOR REMEDY KITS

1. Individual Remedy Kits

Various anthroposophical physicians have developed their own home remedy kits and can advise as to their use. Often recommended remedies are listed on page 13.

2. The Healing Kit

As shown in Sandra Greenstone's Book *Healing at Home*, Healing at Home Resources (see page 11).

> Sprain Care (Arnica Ointment)
> Arnica 6X
> Wound Care (Balsamicum Ointment)
> Carbo Betulae Powder 3X
> Chamomile Flowers— loose biodynamic/organic tea— no tea bags
> Echinacea Compound
> Cinnabar Compound
> Burn Care (Combudoron Gel)
> Eucalyptus Oil
> Infludoron
> Lavender Oil

3. The Absolute Basic Kit

Lioba Logan, a mother of 5, reduced her "home remedy kit" to: Weleda Arnica Massage Oil. Massaging her children's backs kept them going to school without getting sick for years on end. She also kept sage tea for sore throat, and chamomile flowers for a stomachache compress.

4. Travel Kit

Keep in mind what conditions you will most likely encounter *while you travel* and what might you likely encounter *at your destination*.

What to take along

Arnica 6X	Trauma
Arnica Massage Oil	Aches; tiredness
Arnica Ointment	Bruising
Calendula Ointment	Abrasions
Chamomile Tea	Cramps
Chamomile 3X	Stomachaches
Charcoal Tablets	Diarrhea
Cinnabar Comp	Sore Throat
Echinacea Comp	Flu
Ginger	Nausea; Indigestion
Melissengeist	Faintness, Spaciness
Sedative Pilules	Sleeplessness

5. Kitchen Remedies

Sage	Sore Throats
Chamomile	Stomach Upset; Compresses
Ginger	Digestive Complaints; and with honey and lemon for Respiratory Congestion
Horseradish	Sinus Compress
Lemon	Fever, Compress; Wheezing
Onion	Inflammation; Joint Pain
Honey	Sore Throat (raw is best)
Sea Salt	Baths
Frozen Peas	Ice pack (molds perfectly to injury, less cold than ice)

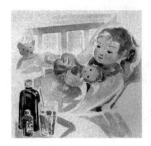

6. A Children's Essential Home Remedy Kit

Arnica 6X Internal — Trauma
Arnica Massage Oil — Warmth (over age 3!)
Arnica Ointment — Bruises
Band Aids, gauze and scissors — Cuts and Scrapes (decorated Band Aids)
Calendula Essence and Ointment — Inflammation; Disinfectant
Chamomile Flowers — Upset Tummies
Combudoron Gel (Burn Care) — Burns and Bites
Compress Cloths
Hot Water Bottle and Thermometer

Moms and Dads

Some tips from parent Mary Carmichael when treating your sick child:
- Forgive yourself when you panic and resort to Tylenol. Reflect on what you could have done differently and talk to others for support.
- Going against the mainstream takes courage, knowledge, and practice.
- Illness helps both the sick and the caregiver. Each grows from a major illness.
- Complementary care becomes a lifestyle, not merely a new form of medicine.
- Convalescent time is critical. It helps prevent relapses and secondary infections or complications. Just realize you'll be home for several days.

The Cocoon

Imagine being a very sick child, and imagine someone taking the time to create a "cocoon" for you to rest and heal in. First you are dressed in warm clothing such as flannel, with a hot water bottle at your feet and a warm, sweet-smelling wrap on the sick area. A warm wool blanket tucks you in, and then you get a good story and some hot tea. Wraps are not just about treatment. Wraps are all about someone taking time to care for you and let you rest. They are about the warmth of love and the warmth of being healed.

COMPRESSES AND POULTICES, SOAKS, WRAPS, AND DEFINITIONS

These are excellent ways to address illnesses through the avenue of the skin. On the following pages we have listed some basic procedures. At first they may seem complicated, but with practice you will find them easy and satisfying. Ask a nurse (see p. 11) to lead you through them first time, or plan a few sessions and practice on one another. Children will enjoy this too; they can practice on their dolls.

1. A **Bath** becomes therapeutic when a medicinal herb or essential oil is added. Temperature too plays an important role.
2. A **Compress** is a natural-fiber cloth saturated with a liquid carrying the substance of a plant or mineral, then folded and either applied directly to the skin or indirectly, with another cloth such a flannel or wool, folded over it.
3. A **Foot Bath** often has the effect of drawing congestion down out of the head or stimulating warmth for the whole body.
4. A **Room Inhalation** is an oil or plant extract placed in the well of a vaporizer or in a bowl on the radiator and allowed to diffuse into the room. (see chamomile, lavender, lemon, eucalyptus).
5. A **Steam Inhalation** is an oil or plant extract in a bowl of hot or boiling water, with a towel or blanket tent over it, and the head placed within the tent. Take care not to get burnt. Keep hair dry to prevent later chilling.
6. A **Poultice** is a natural fiber folded "envelope" holding hot or cool whole or chopped plants or herbs, then applied to the body and covered. See Onion Poultice for earaches (also ginger and mustard poultices).
7. A **Sitz Bath** is a bath where one sits in a basin although the whole body is submerged.
8. A **Soak** is an essence or tea diluted in hot or cool water, submerging a limb. (A hot calendula soak draws splinters, a cool combudoron soak helps alleviate burns. A warm rosemary foot bath helps relieve headaches.)
9. A **Wrap** is a compress which is wrapped all around the body.

1. Baths

Baths are a wonderful way to dispense nature's healing gifts to the body. While pills and other internal remedies work via the metabolism, external treatments affect the body through the nervous system. With baths, compresses and oils—a very large perceptive organ is addressed—the skin. Baths are relaxing, and easy to prepare. They help create a warm and protective environment that is as important as the substances you add. Baths are wonderful even when you are well.

Preparation for most therapeutic baths: Prepare the bed with a pillow, a sheet (preferably flannel), a towel for the head and a towel for the feet (for wrapping), and blankets.
Warmth: The room should be warm and the windows closed.
Considerations: Create a mood that is quiet and concentrated. Avoid conversation, except with children.
Length: In general, the sicker or more delicate the patient, the shorter the bath. Patients who are very ill and weak may not tolerate bath therapy. *Except* for an overwarming sweat bath the patient should get out as soon as there is perspiration on the face.
Frequency: Avoid too frequent or too long baths. Avoid too much external heat, except when using an overwarming bath. The patient should not perspire during the rest period, except with an overwarming bath.
Afterwards: Occasionally a person will feel faint on getting out of the tub, because blood vessels are dilated. Stay with the patient until he or she is safely back in bed.
If a substance is used, wrap the patient loosely, without drying, in a large towel or flannel sheet. Avoid "air holes." Cover the patient with blankets and wrap the head (except for the face) and the shoulders with a towel. Apply a covered warm water bottle under the feet if necessary (see page 79). The caregiver should be available and should periodically assess the patient. Allow plenty of time for rest, usually 30–45 minutes at least.

Aromatic Oil Baths

These baths introduce therapeutic plant oils to the organism by means of the skin. They help in a variety of situations, augmenting plantlike up-building (metabolic) processes. Full immersion, at close to body temperature, encourages "perception" of the substance. **Note:** Make sure the bathroom is warm so no chilling occurs.

Procedure: Fill bathtub with comfortably warm water, a little above body temperature. Add 1–2 teaspoons bath oil or essence of your choice. Water coming out of the pipes is devitalized because of a lack of proper movement. You can enliven the bath water by gently moving it as the tub fills. It is important not to agitate the water but to move it gently in an organized way until it feels light. A figure-eight with emphasis toward the center is a nice way of doing it. Let the water come to rest for a few seconds before the patient enters the bath.

Length: Let the patient rest, immersed in the water for 7–15 minutes. Do not use soap.

Afterwards: Without drying the patient off, wrap quickly in a large towel, and put to bed, wrapping well in a flannel sheet. (Use wrapped warm water bottle for the feet if necessary.) Let the patient rest for 45–60 minutes in a quiet room. Avoid books or TV and let this be a healing time.

Some Popular Bath Oils

Rosemary Bath—an incarnating bath
Pine Bath—refreshing, harmonizing, cleansing; it lets you breathe
Lemon Bath—refreshes and invigorates and gives you a "border"
Lavender Bath—relaxes and helps induce sleep

Arnica Oil Bath for Dry Skin

Procedure: For uncomfortably dry skin, especially in winter, pour a teaspoon of Arnica Massage Oil under the tap of a tub filling with warm water. Stir vigorously to disperse the oil in the water. Soak in the mixture for 10–15 minutes without using soap. Dry gently. The oil should be fully absorbed by the body.

Nutritional Bath

Note: Nutritional Baths are powerful and should not be approached lightly. Please consult your physician if in doubt. Do not administer if there is a fever or evidence of local inflammation (flu, cold, otitis, an inflamed cut, etc.). Do not take during acute illness, or if antibiotics or other medications are being taken.

Before you begin: Prepare the bed, as described in the introduction to baths.

How often: Ideally, nutritional baths are given in a series of 7 (once a week). Give them on the same days of the week at the same time, surrounding them with a peaceful atmosphere, and never fail to provide rest afterwards.

Indications: Convalescence, nutritional disorders, stress, addictions and withdrawal, children who are not "themselves" after an experience or an illness, detoxification after exposure to chemicals or antibiotics, etc.

Temperature: This is a substance bath. Temperature should be only a little above body temperature, preferably not be above 95–98 degrees Fahrenheit, but the patient must be comfortable. Warm the bathroom and the bedroom prior to the treatment.

> **Ingredients:**
> 1 free range or organic egg (yolk used only)
> 1 cup raw cow's milk (or, if not available, at least use non-homogenized, no vitamin A+D milk of the best quality available
> 1 biodynamic or organic lemon
> **Supplies:** small bowl, sharp knife, fork, container for compost

Procedure: Draw the bath water slightly above the desired temperature. Break the egg, separating the yolk—then gently stir the yolk in a bowl, adding the milk, until well mixed. Cut the lemon as described on p. 80 for Lemon Calf Wrap. Add the milk-and-egg mixture to the tub. Mix the ingredients and lighten the water by stirring it in a gentle, organized way. One can use a figure eight motion. Think of weaving two opposite poles together; a picture of the rhythmic system. Keep your movements fluid and avoid splashing water against the ends of the tub, and don't let your attention wander; it will detract from the effectiveness of the bath. The hand should not "cut through" the water but rather draw the water along with it—moving with the water.

The water is then allowed to become quiet. Lay the patient in the water, submerged to the neck for 5–15 minutes. After the bath, wrap the patient as described previously, without drying. The rest period should ideally be one hour. Young children can be put into their pajamas damp (if they are of pure, untreated cotton) and allowed to sleep through the night. Adjust their wrappings after a short time so they do not perspire. It is important to observe for the response, and to do this treatment in a rhythm.

Caution: If the patient shows perspiration on the face, bring him/her out of the bath. Perspiring should also not occur during the rest period. It could undo the effects of the treatment. Loosen wraps as needed to prevent overheating.

Overwarming/Sweat Bath

Indications: If the patient is ill and not running a fever, some of the benefits of fever can be obtained by use of a sweat bath. This bath is also effective in early illness, in helping an illness that is "stuck" to get moving again, or when the patient is bone chilled (except when the chill is due to a rising fever).
Caution: This is only to be used if fever is under 100 degrees Fahrenheit, and is only recommended for young, healthy people with strong hearts.
Procedure: Get into the tub and fill it with water that is a bit hotter than comfortable. Add hot water as needed to maintain the warmth of the bath.
Length: Stay for approximately 15–20 minutes.
Drink plenty of hot liquids while doing this. You need to be hydrated. Dry off and wrap without getting chilled; then rest, or sleep, if possible under warm covers for at least one hour (cover head with a wool hat or towel).

Sitz Bath:
See instructions on pages 62 and 79.

2. Compresses

Arnica Compress *For bruises and sprains.*

Procedure: Dilute one part Arnica Essence to nine parts water, as a cool compress to the forehead or as a compress for bruising. For a sprained ankle take a cool wet arnica compress and cover with a wool wrap. Continue to add moisture under wool wrap. Maintain moist compress until swelling has gone down, then apply Arnica Ointment. Do not apply to open wounds.

Chamomile Abdominal Compress *For infant colic, certain sleep disturbances, menstrual cramps, too much sensory stimulation, inflamed eyes, or overburdened nerves, especially in children, and mild digestive problems.*

Caution: Do *not* use unless a physician approves the use of heat applicaions if there is *any* acute abdominal illness, especially where there is pain and/or fever.
Procedure: See General Compress Procedures. You will need: boiling water; loose chamomile flowers, preferably organic; strainer, silk/cotton wrap & wool wrap, wringing towel (cotton tea towel), and a bowl.

a) Create a scroll as large as the area to be covered, using a cotton inner cloth and a wool outer cloth.
b) Lay the patient over this scroll in preparation.
c) Take a silk or cotton cloth of the appropriate size and fold once or twice to fit the area being treated. Then roll it up loosely.
d) Place rolled cloth inside a folded wringing cloth (and towel).
e) Place approx. 1 heaping teaspoon chamomile flowers in a small saucepan. Pour 3 cups boiling water over them. Allow to steep for 2–3 minutes *maximum*, then strain.
f) Place compress in a bowl so that it fits completely inside and the free ends of the wringing towel are hanging over the edge. Pour hot tea over the package.

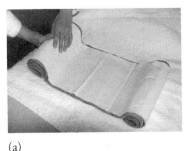

(a)

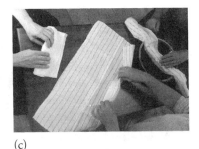

(c)

g) Wring it out as if you were "wringing water from a stone." The more thoroughly you wring it, the better it works.
h) Remove hot compress quickly and "air" briefly over surface of area with hands to avoid burning. Then apply to area. It must give a warmth "surge" when applied or it will not function well. This aspect is very important and difficult to achieve, and should therefore be practiced. If it is not applied hot enough, it will cool too quickly.

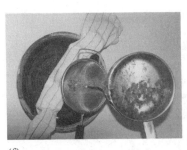

(f)

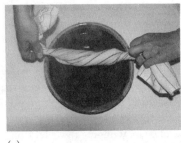

(g)

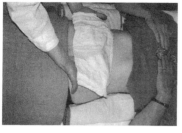

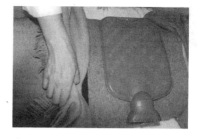

(i)   (j)

i) Wrap scrolled wool compress *rapidly* and securely around abdomen so no air can penetrate to the wet compress.

j) Apply a *flat* hot water bottle (see page 79).

k) Cover patient warmly with a blanket.

l) Leave on for the duration of the treatment (45 minutes to 1 hour), if the compress remains warm. Remove wet compress from under the wool wrap. Leave the wool wrap and hot water bottle in place for another 5–10 minutes until the skin dries, so there is no chilling. If the compress feels cool to the patient at any point in the treatment, remove it immediately from under the wool. Leave the wool and the hot water bottle in place for the whole treatment period. Review your technique, so compress is applied warmer or is maintained warmer next time.

Caution: Be sure no light is shining into patient's eyes. It affects the digestion and the ability to rest.

Eucalyptus Oil Bladder Compress *Adjunctive treatment for urinary tract infections and for spastic bladder conditions.*

Procedure: Saturate a piece of sheeting in Eucalyptus Essential Oil, diluted 1:10 in cold-pressed vegetable oil. Protect it in a plastic bag, and warm it on a hot water bottle. Remove it from the bag. Apply to skin over bladder and cover it with several layers of flannel rags or with a pillow made of cotton batting. Never apply essential oils directly to the skin without first diluting them. Hold this in place over bladder with underpants, and it can be kept on all night.

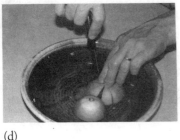
(d)

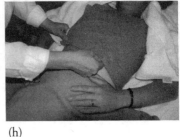
(h)

Hot Lemon Compress *For deep cough, chest congestion, wheezing, bronchitis, bronchial asthma.*

(Weleda's Plantago Ointment is another application for congestion and is suitable for children.)

Procedure: You will need: cotton cloth (wash cloth), lemon, boiling water, knife and fork, wringing cloth (hand towel), warm shirt, and wool blanket. Have everything ready by the bed. If the feet are not warm, use a covered hot water bottle.

a) Scroll the compress cloth.

b) Place inside wringing cloth.

c) Pour boiling water into a medium-size bowl. Let cool 2 minutes.

d) Cut the lemon in half as you would for the lemon calf wrap. Score the skin in the water, using a knife and fork. Then press lemon with the bottom of a jar or glass to release essential oils and juice.

e) Place wringing cloth pack in bowl with ends hanging over the sides. Soak, then remove and wring until dripping stops.

f) Remove compress from inside wringing cloth.

g) Apply compress to the patient's upper chest. It should be as hot as the patient can tolerate but *do not burn.*

h) Quickly wrap wool covering around so that no part of compress peeks out—it would cool too quickly.

i) Cover patient with warm clothes and blanket.

j) Remove compress when no longer hot. Take from under wool covering, leaving wool in place until the skin is dry.

Note: Great care must be taken not to *chill* the patient at any time during this procedure.

Yarrow Compress

Same as for Chamomile Compress, but rectangular compress applied over liver.

3. Foot Baths

Foot baths are an excellent way to warm the body, treat weary feet, and even subdue a headache. Fill a mid-calf-height bucket with warm water (higher for headache relief). Avoid a bucket that was used for detergents or chemicals. Add a teaspoon of the healing substance.

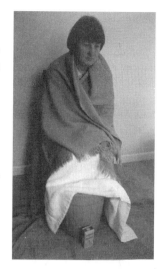

Mustard Foot Bath *Colds and chills; headache relief, head colds.*

Mix a small handful or two of dry mustard in warm water (not hot water; it deactivates mustard). Cover the patient well with towels and have a towel on the floor under the footbath. After the skin is strongly stimulated, usually 15–20 minutes, rinse the feet and calves well with a pitcher of warm water. Be sure you rinse between the toes. Mustard baths are an excellent way to draw an illness out.

Rosemary Foot Bath *Relieves headache.*

1–2 teaspoons added to enough warm water to cover feet and ankles. This foot bath is also helpful for the elderly or bedridden to help wake up in the morning, and to stimulate the circulation in the lower extremities.

Lemon Foot Bath *Hay fever, headache, sinus, flu, before or after a fever (not during), bronchitis; and those times when a child needs "bringing back in"; clearing the head and connecting with the more physical nature. It also has healing benefits for cases of depression and fatigue.*

Its properties are warmth, light, order, vitality, contraction (due to its sourness), and form (due to its shape and inner construction). Prepare as for Lemon Calf Wraps, in warm water.

4. Inhalations

Chamomile Inhalation *To loosen congestion (bronchitis), soothe membranes of the nose and oropharynx, open plugged eustachian tubes with ear*

infections, and speed healing of a cold.

Procedure: Put a small handful of loose chamomile flowers in the bottom of a mixing bowl and pour boiling water over them. Place on a low table. Sit patient at table, warmly dressed and with a hot water bottle at feet if necessary. Cover hair with a towel or shower cap so there's no chilling after. Drape another large towel over head and bowl to create a tent. Steam should be slowly but deeply inhaled through nose and mouth. Repeat procedure, if needed to maintain steam, for 15–20 minutes. Repeat as necessary. Be careful not to burn. For children try building a large tent with a blanket and make a game of it. Join them inside. Afterwards, dry the patient's face, apply a warm hat, and ensure a quiet time of at least half an hour. *Never leave young children unattended with this.*

Eucalyptus Room or Steam Inhalation

Procedure: Sprinkle a few drops of Eucalyptus Oil in lukewarm water and place on radiator, or add to hot steam vaporizer. You can also use Rosemary, Lavender, or other oils.

Lavender Room Inhalation
For relief of stress put Lavender Oil or Lavender Bath in a bowl on the radiator, or into the vaporizer.

Lemon Room Inhalation
Cut and score a lemon under lukewarm water to preserve all essential oils, and place in water on radiator.

5. Poultices

Chamomile Poultice *Especially good for the abdomen.*

Procedure: Take a handful of chamomile flowers (2 tablespoons) and put in bottom of saucepan. Pour boiling water on; enough to soak. Cover, let steep a maximum of 3 minutes. Empty onto a tea towel or compress cloth and proceed as with compress.

Ginger Sinus Poultice *For sinus infections.*

Caution: Not for hay-fever, simple head colds, etc. Be careful! Ginger can burn.
Procedure: You will need fresh ginger root (rhizome), a grater, teaspoon,

a cotton sheet, a wool blanket, facial tissue, lanolin or petroleum jelly.

a) Bring ingredients to the bedside and drape patient with sheet and blanket.

b) Put a warm water bottle wrapped in a towel at the feet (feet must be warm while receiving this treatment).

c) Grate the ginger root very fine. Or use ginger powder.

d) For each poultice mix about 1/2 teaspoon powder well to make a thick paste.

e) Spoon onto the center of each poultice cloth and fold over to make a package. Tape the edges if you like.

f) Fold 2 rectangles of facial tissue about 1 1/2 inches and apply jelly (not petroleum) to one side.

g) With clean fingers, apply the tissues with the jelly side down to both eyes. Stroke downward over the closed eyes to seal the lashes. Covering the eyes helps prevent the strong vapors from irritating them.

h) Apply poultices over the sinuses, and have the patient hold them until a pink area develops on the skin that is even in color and the same size as the compresses. Then remove the compresses.

Caution: Leaving poultices on too long can cause blisters.

i) Apply oil (e.g., olive oil) on the area.

j) Remove the used tissues and wipe eyes clean with a new one.

k) Have the patient rest for at least 45 minutes to 1 hour after the treatment. Treatment may be repeated once a day if the skin tolerates this.

Mustard Poultice *For the chest* (see instructions for ginger poultice).

Procedure: Bring all the ingredients to the bedside and drape patient with a sheet and blanket. Secure hot water bottle at feet with towel. (Feet must be warm while receiving this treatment.)

a) Spread mustard powder on poultice cloth, about 1/8–1/4 inch thick.

b) Fold into an envelope and pin it closed. Roll it gently into a loose cylinder.

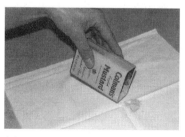 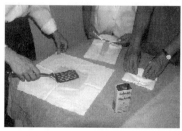

(a)   (b)

c) Dip and wet in warm (not hot) water. When saturated, gently press (without wringing) to express excess water.

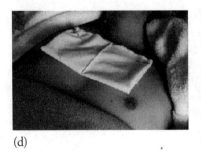
(d)

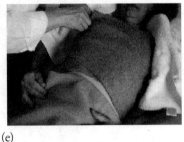
(e)

d and e) Open and apply to chest and cover quickly with wool.

Remove the compress when a smooth pink area develops that is the same size as the compress. (If you are doing this for yourself, set an alarm clock or timer for 15 minutes to prevent you burning yourself if you fall asleep.) Have the patient rest for at least 45 minutes to 1 hour after the treatment. Treatment may be repeated as often as once a day if the skin tolerates this. Otherwise skip a day between treatments.

Caution: Leaving compress on too long can cause blisters. Put oil on area.

Onion Poultice *Organizes the inflammation of an earache. Also helps release fluid caused by allergies.*

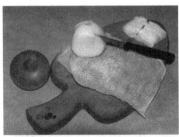

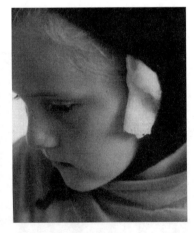

This is very effective in loosening painful congestion in the ear, just as an onion draws tears from the eyes. A number of different variations for applying warm, raw, cut up, yellow or white onions will work. You can use onion juice expressed with a garlic press on a cotton ball warmed and placed in the outer ear.

Remember: It is important to keep the ear and entire head warm. Keep a wool stocking cap pulled over both ears. Make sure the onion is always warmed before putting it on the ear. A hot water bottle does well for this.

6. Sitz Baths

Eucalyptus Sitz Bath *For yeast infections* (see page 62).

Fill a small bottle or jar 1/3 with water. Put 1–2 capfuls of Eucalyptus Essential Oil in the jar and shake vigorously to disperse it in the water. Draw the bath as warm as tolerated and as high as the navel and pour the oil mixture into the running water. Sit for about 15 minutes with a towel over the shoulders. Don't use soap. After the bath, dry off very carefully, wrap warmly, and rest for 30–45 minutes (may be done at bedtime).

Vinegar Sitz Bath *For yeast infections* (see page 62).

Add 1 tablespoon vinegar to 1/2 tub warm water. Dry off very carefully— you might even use a hair dryer on a low setting.

7. Soaks

Calendula Soak *Inflammations, abrasions.*

Dilute 1 part Calendula Essence to 9 parts water as a cool or tepid compress or wash. Use as a hot soak for boils or to help draw splinters.

Procedure for a Warm Water Bottle

Fill hot water bottle a third full with hot tap water (you may add a little boiling water to this if tap water is not hot enough). Expel all the air from the bottle to the point where water enters the neck of the bottle, and tightly screw on the cap. Cover with a wool cloth for extra protection.

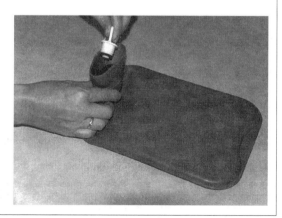

---

8. Wraps

Arnica Calf and Foot Wrap *To warm the feet, especially for the elderly.*
Caution: Never apply direct heat to feet if circulation is poor.
Add two capfuls Arnica Essence to 3 cups warm water. Wrap calves and feet
as for Lemon Calf Wraps.

Combudoron Wrap *For minor burns.*
Caution: Before wrapping, immediately soak for 15 minutes in cool water.
Then create a wrapped compress.
Procedure: You will need Combudoron Burn Care Gel, a cotton/linen sterile wrap or sterile gauze squares; roll gauze if needed.
a) Be sure hands and equipment are clean.
b) Soak compress in body-temperature or cool water. Wring out so it is moist but not dripping.
c) Spread a thick layer of Burn Care Gel onto the cloth. The compress must never dry. Add water to keep it moist.
d) Lightly wrap around burn area, making sure there are no air holes.

Eucalyptus Oil Bladder Wrap—see Compresses

Lemon Calf and Foot Wrap *To gently reduce and organize a fever response.*
Caution: Do not use with cold feet or if there is no fever. Feet *must* be warm prior to treatment. Have all materials ready. Patient should be dressed warmly and covered. Protect the bed under the calves and feet with a towel.
Procedure: You will need a lemon, preferably organic, a bowl (glass or pottery), a knife, warm water, 2 cotton wraps (about 6 inches longer than the person is tall; 4 inches wide for children and 6 inches wide for adults), 2 same size wool wraps or long wool socks.
a) Roll up wraps loosely from one end and have them ready at hand.
b) Place lemon in bowl and pour warm water over it.
c) Cut the lemon underwater in the following way: Cut in half, with the flat sides on the bottom of the bowl, slice each as you would a cake (in wedges) half leaving the core intact. Score the skin all over (make little cuts with a sharp knife) to release oil from the skin. Then express the juice.

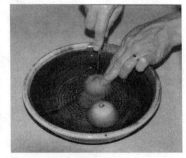

d) Soak the cotton wraps in the lemon water.

e) Wring out one wrap at a time as well as you can.

f) Apply the wrap to one leg, starting at the toes and moving up just below to the knee.

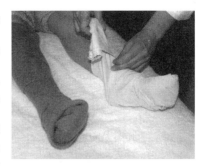

g) Immediately, apply the wool wrap in the same manner on top of the cotton wrap, covering the wet wrap completely.

h) Cover patient. Be sure that no open spaces are left in either wrap. The skin should be covered from the tips of the toes nearly to the knees with the cotton wrap, and the cotton should be completely covered with the firm wool wrapping.

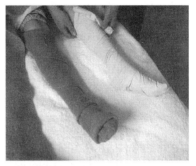

Check cotton wrap after 15 minutes:

If dry, remove and apply freshly dipped wrap.

If cool, remove and redo. Be sure that there are no leaks in the wrap, the feet are warm and the wrap is not too wet.

If warm and moist, leave on for another 5–10 minutes.

Important: Patient must rest after completion of wraps, protected from drafts in a secure, quiet space. Wraps may be repeated for up to one hour, although this is rarely necessary.

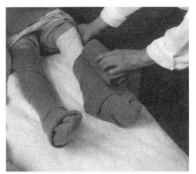

Lemon Throat Wrap *For sore throat in older children and adults.*

a) Prepare same as for chest wrap. Proceed as above, but apply to the neck.

b) Use cotton/wool wraps sized for the patient's neck.

CARING FOR THE PATIENT WITH FEVER

by Margaret Rosenthaler, RN

After years of encouraging the use of aspirin and Tylenol even "regular medicine" is slowly learning that it is usually best to let patients have their fevers. But as we bravely try to carry out this resolve, we are plagued by spectres planted in our thoughts and feelings.

In nursing and medical schools we learn (and teach our patients, too) to immediately look for the "worst case scenario." Of the child who has a fever, we say, "His temperature could go so high it could destroy his brain." This way of thinking causes us to fear such challenging episodes. A certain zone of comfort for the caregiver is reached by eliminating the fever and by preventing "any possibility of injury."

Now we learn that in order to pass through many illnesses successfully and completely the patient needs a fever. Repeated suppression of acute illness often leads to chronic debility. The importance of febrile illness in promoting the remodeling of the body, and the flexibility of normal growth and development, are forfeited if fevers and inflammations are repeatedly suppressed.

How then can we help a sick person to go through a fever in a good way? To begin to understand this, we need to comprehend a little better how warmth works in the body. In the mineral and plant world temperatures tend to even out and to achieve a certain uniformity; in the human organism warmth varies from one part of the body to another. The liver, for example, is always in a kind of fever, warmth being essential for all metabolic activity. Muscles become warm with exercise and need warmth for proper function. One can damage muscles by using them rigorously when they are cold. On the other hand the nervous system, especially the head, needs to be cool. Remember how your head felt on a day when it was exposed to too much sun? It ached, and thinking was especially difficult. A "hot-headed" person is not particularly a philosopher. When someone is thinking clearly, we say that he has a "cool head." In general there is a polarity operating between the upper and the lower parts of our organism, the upper needing to be cooler, the lower requiring warmth (the abdomen and the limbs). This polarity is especially important for the proper functioning of the organism. And unlike our immediate surroundings, in health our body can regulate its overall temperature and temperature of its organs.

This polarity must be maintained even during fever. Some people are better at this than others and are able to tolerate higher temperatures with fewer ill effects. Others are less successful and tend to suffer more during fever (e.g.

headache, delirium, achiness, restlessness, lethargy, increased sensitivity.) There-fore, in treating fever, it is important to support this polarity by keeping the head cool and the rest of the body warm. Wrap the patient warmly he/she is working hard to raise his/her temperature. Administer only warm or room tem-perature food and fluids. (Cooling the abdomen pushes warmth into the head, reversing the polarity.) Lemon foot and calf wraps are very effective in restoring disturbed polarity; they divert warmth from the head. They should only be applied if the feet are warm. If the feet are cool, rub them gently or apply a covered hot water bottle. An older patient might need an Arnica Essence Calf and Foot Wrap to warm the feet prior to applying the Lemon Calf and Foot Wraps (see page 80). Never apply direct heat to feet where the circulation is poor or the feeling is impaired (e.g., diabetes and the elderly).

Other measures can be taken to help fever run a healthy course. Much of it is traditional knowledge, lost in recent years. Fever essentially creates a lot of debris or waste which must be expelled from the body to prevent complications. Care needs to be taken to see that the patient has three loose stools per day. It is amazing to see how much patients with fever can elimi-nate even when they are not eating.

Urea is a major by-product of tissue destruction, and urea levels as well as the level of other waste products in the blood rise with fever. This is responsible for a lot of the discomfort (malaise) and neurologic irritability during fever, since urea is neurotopic. Urine is often dark in color because the increased waste is being cleared from the system. Encouraging a high intake of warm or room-tempera-ture fluids helps clean the blood and protects kidneys stressed by fever.

The increased urea in the blood has another aspect. How does eating protein affect a person with a fever? Their body is in a catabolic state, and not particularly inclined to build up tissue. Protein eaten during a fever is mostly broken down and just adds to the toxic burden of urea in the blood. It is best to provide meals free of protein, if the patient wishes to eat at all. Grains, vegetables, and fruits can be given. Don't be surprised by weight loss during fever. It is part of the process.

Because the nerves are irritable from the increased warmth of the body, and as a result of the high waste levels in the blood and tissues, it is impor-tant to protect the nervous system and the senses. The environment should be quiet, the lights low. Pictures that could provide a stimulus for fevered nightmares and delirium should be removed from the walls and the room should be clean and orderly to balance the inner disturbance that the pa-tient experiences. Radio, electronic games, and TV are detrimental during fever, because the severe stress they place on the nerves can predispose the patient to neurological complications.

It is important to have access to medical assessment and advice with all of the above, so seek out a physician who is supportive of your philosophy of treatment.

DIET
Life in the Balance by Louise Frazier

If we consider the human organism as constantly in a state of seeking balance—how can nutrition best be applied? Of course nutrition is in the frontline of prevention, as many studies show today.

To begin with we can weave a measure of harmony by eating foods of our bioregion in all its seasons. This has the effect of connecting us with the in-breathing and out-breathing of the earth where we live and breathe. Relief from functioning with an organism designed for a different section of our country or even another part of the world with today's food supply is to our benefit. Considering pollution as a major factor in creating a toxic environment, eating food grown closer to home instead of trucked from far and wide also makes sense. Most important to protect us from the many manipulations by the food industry, with all their unknown effects, is to choose biodynamic/organic foods. The earth in its natural state is able to team up with healing, life-giving forces instead of losing itself in chemicals and excess water.

Priest-King Zarathustra, who guided ancient human beings into cultivation of the land, knew that cosmic forces in the sun rayed into the grains grown in the fields. He saw this effect radiating into the human being when ingesting the fruit of the grain harvest, leading people to pause and to imagine: "the Sun will rise in you when you enjoy the fruits of the field." That nourishment is still available to us today through biodynamic/organic agricultural practices. Steaming dishes of rice, sunny millet, barley, and oats are foods to nurture the hale and hearty, as well as the frail and ill. Young or old can experience enveloping warmth, balance, and strength in simple or grand whole-grain foods.

Many people were restored to health through the work of Werner Kollath, the German medical doctor and nutritionist. He fed them a diet based on fresh grains, especially wheat berries cracked in a heavy old coffee grinder. Soaking the grains in water for 5–10 hours and adding grated apples or other fruit, raisins, nuts, and honey created a miracle food. Research showed his fresh-grain "muesli" to have regenerative qualities. A similar breakfast can be made easily by soaking overnight third of a cup of organic steel-cut oats in a bowl with half a cup of fresh cold water topped with a saucer and set aside on the counter at room temperature. In the morning, add grated or chopped fresh fruits or whole berries of the season, or soaked dried organic fruits such as apples, apricots, pears, along with 1 Tbs each of sunflower seeds or chopped nuts, raisins, fresh lemon juice, and 1 tsp of honey, if desired. All the better if one has a grain mill and can grind the grains fresh each time.

Louise's Leaves by **Louise Frazier**. This guide to year-round cooking for flavor and nutrition celebrates the seasons and local vegetables. The author has many years' experience in biodynamic/organic gourmet food preparation: 86 pp., $9.75. Biodynamic Farming and Gardening Association, PO Box 29135, San Franicsco, CA 94129-0135. Tel: (888) 516-7797.

A Daily Health Menu

From: *Diet and Cancer*, U. Renzenbrink, Anthroposophic Press (p. 11).

Breakfast
1. "Muesli" (p. 84) with soured milk *or* freshly ground grains soaked overnight, cooked in the same water and left to absorb the moisture. Add the same ingredients.
2. Whole-grain bread, butter with quark* or cheese or (if sweetness is craved) fruit concentrates or honey. An apple or fruit in season.
3. Herb tea.

Lunch
1. Cup of vegetable broth, tea, or warmed lactic fermented vegetable juice.
2. Raw vegetables or salad.
3. Grain dishes, alternating each day, matched with cooked or raw vegetables. Sauces made with herbs. If desired and suitable a milk pudding, quark* dessert or stewed fruit.

Evening Meals
1. Soup made with freshly ground grains and herbs or stewed dried fruits.
2. Soured milk products such as buttermilk or kefir.
3. Bread, butter, light cheeses, herb tea.
   Between meals: herb tea, crisp bread, wholemeal biscuits, fruit, nuts, honey, fruit juices, soured milk products, lactic fermented vegetable juice.

Recipes for Use with Weleda Tonics (see page 87)

Celeriac/Apple Salad: Season one cup cottage cheese with celery salt, lemon juice, and a little mustard. Add 2 tablespooons Blackthorn Tonic and quickly mix in one grated apple and half a celeriac, also grated.

Cottage Cheese/Grapefruit Salad: On a bed of lettuce arrange cottage cheese and grapefruit pieces. Top with a yogurt-cream dressing, seasoned with mustard, salt and 2 tablespoons Blackcurrent Tonic. Add cut fruit to yogurt. Top with 1 tablespoon Blackthorn Tonic.

Frozen Yogurt: Mix yogurt and Blackthorn or Blackcurrant Tonic to taste and freeze for one hour, stir down and refreeze for 30 minutes.

*Quark is a soured milk product (*fromage frais*). You can easily make it at home by suspending yogurt in a muslin bag until the whey has run out.

Diet During Illness

With any type of inflammation, cold, or fever, eating less is better than eating more. When your body is trying to "digest" and eliminate toxic substances it helps if you don't have to digest too much at once. Avoid *protein foods* (meat, eggs, dairy, nuts, fish) and *legumes* (beans, peas, lentils, soy) during acute illness. Give mainly a liquid diet of vegetable broth, herb teas and fruit juices, but no colder than room temperature. Fruit, cooked vegetables, grains, and light crackers are suitable.

The return of appetite is a sign of getting better, but those first meals after the fever is down should be light. Don't be too eager to have your children regain the lost weight, although they might be ravenous. After the illness, reintroduce the restricted foods gradually and carefully.

Vegetable Soup

Keep a soup stock on hand made with fresh organic or preferably biodynamic vegetables. Use potatos, carrots, a few green beans, squash, or spinach. Add peas for interest and parsley or other herbs to taste. Use braised onion or garlic only if the patient can tolerate it, and add an organic vegetable bouillon if you want added flavor. Salt moderately. Simmer for 20 minutes. Serve either with the cut vegetables left in, pureed, or strained and served as a drink. The stock will keep, refrigerated, for one or two days. Onion or garlic or pepper added to the soup add warmth and are good for colds. So do ginger and herbs such as basil, sage, thyme, marjoram, oregano.

KITCHEN REMEDIES
by Marina Poliakoff, The Hungry Hollow Co-op

Horseradish with Lemon Juice *for nasal congestion.* Chop, grate or process about 1 inch of fresh horseradish, as fine as you can. Start by taking 1/4 teaspoon with a few drops of lemon juice on it. Chew very well before swallowing. Increase to 1/2 teaspoon twice daily between meals.

Onion and Honey Remedy *for cough.* Grate a small onion in a bowl and add the same amount of raw honey (it must be raw). Mix well and eat a teaspoon at a time on an empty stomach.

Ginger Tea *for nausea, poor digestion, excess mucus.* To one cup of your favorite herb tea, add a few drops of freshly squeezed ginger juice. The juice can be gotten by grating and mashing fresh ginger root.

Licorice Tea *for fatigue, constipation, chest colds.* Bring to a boil 2 cups of water with 2 licorice sticks (root) in it. Simmer 15 minutes. Strain and drink.

WELEDA TONICS

An alternative to vitamin pills

The potent berries, fruits, and leaves used in Weleda tonics are harvested in their natural habitat and grown without pesticides or fertilizers. They are allowed to sun-ripen to full maturity. Their juices are extracted with a special "warming" process, and organic beet sugar is added to preserve them. Fruit tonics are potent, and they are delicious.

Birch Tonic: As we get older our body tends to retain more deposits. Birch is a remedy made of young vital birch leaves. It helps elimination. This is a spring and fall tonic for people over 35.

Blackcurrant Tonic: This is a wonderful digestive aid, especially with heavy meals.

Blackthorn Tonic: Blackthorn (sloe) helps rebuild vital forces after illness or stress.

Elder Tonic: This tonic is made with biodynamic hawthorne flowers and berries. It has a warming effect and helps keep our watery processes flowing, especially as a preventative in colds or the flu.

Sea Buckthorn Tonic: This is a true winter strengthener, especially when resistance is low.

All tonics are taken 2–3 times daily, two to three teaspoons in a glass of hot or room temperature (spring) water. All tonics are great on hot oatmeal or yogurt.

Here are some suggestions for adding variety to these tonics: peppermint tea goes well with Birch or Blackthorn; appleblossom, malva or raspberry leaf teas are enhanced by Blackthorn; lemon Melissa or linden teas by Sea Buckthorn.

HERBAL TEAS

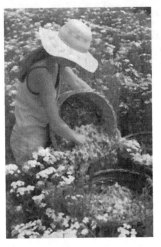

A wonderful way to receive a plant's healing gifts is through teas. Extracting the plant's beneficial qualities requires various methods of heating the herb in water. Teas can be made from flowers, leaves, coarse leaves, seeds, and roots or bark. Generally, the more delicate the plant part (the flowers). the less time it needs, while the more substantial part (the root) needs more time. In addition, because everyone is different, each tea will be experienced differently: strongly, more subtly, or as having no effect at all, depending on the person.

Teas for drinking should be light and "fine," giving a clear impression of the plant. On the other hand, teas for external use may be allowed to cook or brew a little longer and may be more concentrated.

Avoid using water from the hot water tap as it is even more devitalized than water from the cold water tap. Good spring or well water is preferable. Most teas must be prepared immediately before use (especially aromatic ones). Do not use aluminum pots.

Instructions for Preparation

1) **Flowers and delicate, aromatic leaves:** Pour boiling water on tea; cover tightly; let stand one minute; strain through a fine sieve.
2) **Tender leaves:** Same procedure as 1), but allow to steep 2–3 minutes.
3) **Thick leaves:** Put tea in saucepan with cold water; cover; bring to a boil; allow to simmer on low heat for 5 minutes; strain.
4) **Aromatic fruits and seeds:** Boil water; add seeds; cover; allow to simmer on low heat for 3-5 minutes; remove from heat; allow to steep 10–15 minutes.
5) **Roots and bark:** Soak in cold water overnight (not in an iron vessel) covered; bring to boil and simmer for 5–10 minutes; strain. You will generally need to stir the tea before using.

TEA CHART

Choose among these for your medicine chest.

TEA	INDICATION
Birch Leaf	A spring cleanser
Chamomile	Stomach, eye compress
Chicory	Bitter
Elder Flower	Sinusitis, Flu
Fennel Seed	Intestinal gas, colic
Ginger	Digestion, Sinus
Horsetail (Equisetum)*	Blood and liver cleanser
Lactagogue Tea	Milk formation
Lemon Balm	Sinusitis
Lemon & Honey	Sore throat and colds
Linden Tea	Colds, sweat inducer
Melissa	Warms stomach, liver
Peppermint	Sinusitis, stomach
Psyllium seed	Laxative
Raspberry Leaf	Menstrual cramps
Rose Hips	Vitamin C, flu
Sage	Sore throat
Sytra Tea	Cough
Sonio Tea	Sleeplessness
Thyme	Laryngitis
Triplex Tea	Stomach tea

Approximate amounts**

To drink—about 1/4 teaspoon per cup
For compresses—1–2 teaspoons to 1/2–3/4 quart water
For wraps—1 "flat" tablespoon to 3/4 quart water
For a bath—1 good handful

Whenever possible, use plants grown biodynamically, or organically. Better still, grow some of your own herbs; harvest and dry them for tea. This is a science and an art in itself.
*no more than 2 cups/day for regular use
**general rules—there are notable exceptions

RESOURCES

Anthroposophical Therapies
(practiced in conjunction with a licensed medical professional.)

Nursing
Anthroposophical nursing extends the traditional art and science of nursing to reflect a more complete picture of the developing human being. Anthroposophical nurses recognize the human being as a spiritual being in a human body. They walk with patients on their unique journey toward healing and know that the healing process ultimately rests within each individual. A course of study for registered nurses is available. Rise Smythe-Freed, RN, Tel: (303) 777-0934.

Therapeutic Eurythmy: Healing Through Movement
Eurythmy is an art of movement that brings the inner dynamics of speech and music to expression through movement and gesture. Its branch, therapeutic eurythmy, is an essential component of anthroposophically extended medicine. It allows the individual to actively participate in the prevention and treatment of illness. Therapeutic eurythmy is an uplifting and inspiring patient resource. Ann Cook, Tel: (707) 568-4288.

Rhythmical Massage
Understanding that rhythm brings healing, this massage was developed in the 1920s by Dr. Ita Wegman, who refined elaborate qualities of touch. enhancing the forces of lightness and levity through lifting and suction. At times when the pressures of life and illness weigh people down, the rhythmic, delicate quality of this form of treatment is a great help. Tel: (610) 469-9689.

Music as Healer
The task of music as healer is to rekindle the memory of the tonal world from which we all were formed. In learning to listen actively and to create sounds, the patient is led into his/her own deeper beingness. For this the lyre, a string instrument, is ideally suited. With simple exercises the music therapist creates a healing atmosphere, gradually fulfilling the silent longing to be in harmony with one's body and with the world. Channa Seidenberg, Tel: (518) 672-4389.

Artistic Therapy
Goethe describes color as movement and activity arising where light and darkness meet. Light and darkness are reflections of the human being—the light of the ego meeting the darkness of substance. In diagnostic drawing and painting, done in a supportive setting, light, darkness, and color becomes outer representations revealing inner movement. It can become an important part of healing. Phoebe Alexander, Tel: (212) 744-0257.

Creative Speech
A pioneering approach that accesses the health-giving, revitalizing forces inherent in the spoken word. Judith Pownal, Tel: (312) 565-2477

Anthroposophical Society: for general resource information. Tel: (734) 662-9355.

Camphill Association of America: For individuals in need of special care. Tel: (610) 469-6162.

Color-Space: Therapeutic living space treatments. Tel: (413) 528-3524.

Danish Imports: Tel: (262) 249-0719.

Flexible Footwear: Tel: (888) 221-7463.

Gradalis Counseling Services: Tel: (303) 448-9124.

New Century Paints: Non-toxic wall paint. Tel: (413) 528-4319.

Lilling: Natural wool clothing. Tel: (800) 747-WOOL.

Morning Rose: Children's woolens. Tel: (877) 686 8200.

Peat Health: Computer protective clothing. Tel: (805) 684-9973

Physicians Association for Anthroposophical Medicine: Tel: (734) 662-1727.

Rose Lyre Workshop: Musical Instruments. Tel: (888) 650-4050.

School of Spiritual Psychology: Tel: (413) 528-3030.

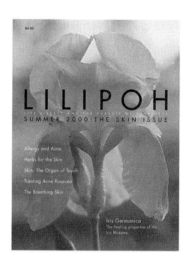

LILIPOH is the journal from which much of the material in this book was taken. Each issue is devoted to a specific theme wherein commonly encountered conditions are addressed by our writers—doctors, nurses, therapists, pharmacists, and lay persons—in a breadth of provocative articles simply written. Besides, there are articles on self-help, biodynamics and nutrition, a parent's and kid's section, political/ rights news, the stars, resources, and more. LILIPOH is available by subscription.

For more information call:
(845) 268-2627,
fax (845) 268-2764,
or write PO Box 649,
Nyack, NY 10977.

www. lilipoh.com
email: info@lilipoh.com

INDEX of MATERIALS and SUBSTANCES

T–Y